OVERCOMING OVEREATING

JANE R. HIRSCHMANN
and CAROL H. MUNTER

Overcoming Overeating

Conquer Your Obsession With Food

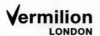
Vermilion
LONDON

In memory of Murry Weiss
C.H.M.

To Edith Schwartz
J.R.H.

*To all those who've had the courage to challenge
the status quo in order to make significant
changes. And with the hope that many more
will do the same.*

First published in the UK 1989
by Heinemann Kingswood

9 11 12 10

Copyright © Jane R. Hirschmann and Carole H. Munter 1988

This edition published in 2000 by Vermilion, an imprint of Ebury Press,
Random House, 20 Vauxhall Bridge Road, London SW1V 2SA

www.randomhouse.co.uk

Random House Australia (Pty) Limited
20 Alfred Street, Milsons Point, Sydney,
New South Wales 2061, Australia

Random House New Zealand Limited
18 Poland Road, Glenfield, Auckland 10, New Zealand

Random House (Pty) Limited
Isle of Houghton, Corner of Boundary Road & Carse O'Gowrie,
Houghton 2198, South Africa

The Random House Group Limited Reg. No. 954009

Papers used by Vermilion are natural, recyclable products made from wood
grown in sustainable forests.

A CIP catalogue record for this title
is available from the British Library
ISBN 9780091825614 (from Jan 2007)
ISBN 009182561X

Printed and bound by
Antony Rowe Ltd, Chippenham, Wiltshire

Contents

THE PLAN: PHASE 3
Finding Yourself

Foreword

Despite the entrenchment of the "diet mentality" in our culture, the past decade has seen the beginnings of yet another revolution in thinking about eating, weight, and dieting. In *Overcoming Overeating*, Jane Hirschmann and Carol Munter present the outline of a program derived from their extensive clinical experience. This program, happily, corresponds in many ways to the sorts of conclusions that basic researchers like us have drawn about the problem of overeating and how to overcome it.

How is this book revolutionary? Readers will be pardoned for being a little cynical at this point, since they have read so many other books, each based on a "revolutionary" premise, promising to help them cope with their weight-and-eating problem. Each of these diet books claims to be "revolutionary" in the sense that it presents a painless, easy shortcut to weight loss, taking advantage of some "secret principle" of nutrition or pattern of eating that allows dieters to overcome the obstacles that have sabotaged all their previous diet efforts. Although these "secret principles" vary from fad to fad, what remains the same are the basic premises: you have to find a way of achieving negative energy balance, that is, expending more calories than you take in, in order to lose weight.

The "secret principles" of successful dieting are not revolutionary; at best, they are seemingly clever tactics that we may employ, invariably without success, in our rebellion against our own weight and eating habits. *Overcoming Overeating is* revolutionary because it challenges the very premises rather than the tactics, of the struggle.

Hirschmann and Munter start with the implicit premise that the problem is overeating, not overweight. This is a significant departure from previous thinking in a couple of respects. First, it implies that we identify our problem behaviorally, not in terms of our appearance. What disturbs Hirschmann and Munter, and their patients, is the compulsive eating in which so many of us engage despite our best intentions. They focus on our obsession with food, our dissatisfaction with our eating habits—we are dissatisfied when we eat and dissatisfied when we don't eat—our guilt, and our sense of being out of control. Their goal is to make us feel better about ourselves, to free us from our compulsive-eating patterns, to achieve some harmony with our bodies—and not simply to lose weight, no matter what it takes.

The second implication in the phrase "overcoming overeating" is that we should not be concerned with devising a plan to ensure successful *under*eating (or a negative energy balance). Rather, if we can eliminate overeating—eating in excess of our bodies' natural requirements—we will have solved the problem. The problem is not overweight but overeating.

But what about overweight? This "problem" may be addressed in a number of ways. For one thing, most dieters are not significantly overweight. Dieting has become so much a part of our culture that women do it regardless of their actual weight, on the assumption that no matter what they weigh, it would be better to weigh less. Second, the evidence points more and more to the conclusion that the alleged health risks of overweight are as much a matter of rapid weight change as of overweight per se. Rapid weight loss is a health

hazard, but so is rapid weight gain, and the dangers of over-weight per se are not as clear to health researchers as they once were. Finally, and most important, dieting causes over-eating. This is the truly revolutionary premise that has emerged in the research literature in the past decade. Clinicians such as Hirschmann and Munter have simultaneously reached the same conclusion on the basis of their exposure to eating-disordered clients. The "compulsive eating" that plagues their clients is eating that is out of sync with the body's natural needs; it is eating for all the wrong reasons. And how does such compulsive eating—more often than not compulsive overeating that produces the dreaded positive energy balance—arise? Almost invariably, it is the result of dieting.

Dieting as we currently define it involves restricting one's intake. This may involve particular classes of food or just overall calories. It may involve severe restrictions—all the way down to protein-supplemented fasts—or just mild de-privations. What all dieting requires, though, regardless of the particulars, is that the dieter learn to give precedence to what the diet allows over what the body demands. (Of course, if the body demanded only what the diet allowed, there'd be no need for dieting.) The crucial problem with all restrictive dieting is that it drives a wedge between a person and his or her body; a struggle ensues, and generally the situation deteriorates. By the time the battle is fully engaged, the dieter, successful or not, has mangled the natural connection between eating and the body's natural signals, since these signals are what the diet is designed to overcome.

Instead of eating on the basis of natural hunger and satiety cues, we eat on the basis of caloric calculations or abstruse nutrient combinations. And what is more ominous, we find ourselves eating on the basis of events not mentioned in our diet charts. Emotional swings of all sorts seem to precipitate disastrous binges, and for some reason, emotional swings seem to increase in frequency and amplitude when we diet. When we start on a treat, allowed by our diet or not, we find it almost impossible to stop. Our eating seems more and more to be under the control of events or stimuli that are inappropriate by any standard, and eventually it seems to be out of control altogether. The compulsive eater eats on the basis of compulsions, mysterious urges to eat that correspond neither to the original hunger (or specific appetites) that are entirely natural nor even to the diet that we substituted for natural eating.

Compulsive eating ruins our eating patterns; more often than not, it ends up increasing our weight, and inevitably, it undermines our sense of self-control and self-esteem. How do we stop the insidious process? First, we must give up dieting as we know it; even "sensible dieting" is a contradiction in terms. But stopping dieting is not enough, particularly if one has lost touch with one's bodily self as a result of extensive dieting. *Overcoming Overeating* provides *practical* guidance to people who are fed up with feeling bad about their eating habits and themselves. This is no mean achievement.

Although researchers have been moving toward a realization of the disruptive and demoralizing effects of dieting, there has been very little in the way of guidance to the individual who wants to quit. Our own book, *Breaking the Diet Habit*, presented all the reasons for quitting but did not provide a comprehensive plan for doing so. Hirschmann and Munter, having worked for so long with so many patients suffering from the compulsive-eating syndrome, have evolved a set of easily understandable and easily applied exercises. Basically, they focus on returning eating to its natural place in one's life, as something to be enjoyed rather than feared, and on improving one's self-concept so that one's problems are dealt with directly rather than compounded by mismanagement through compulsive overeating.

It is not necessary at this point to preview their methods, but it is worth remarking on the pervasive common sense that infuses this book. What is truly remarkable about Hirschmann and Munter's approach is their concern for the problems faced by the compulsive eater, including those posed by letting go of compulsive eating. This book is full of truly practical advice; not only do Hirschmann and Munter make dozens of worthwhile suggestions, but they _integrate_ their suggestions into a complete package that involves both learning to eat appropriately and learning to put eating into an appropriate place in one's life. And not only do they make valuable suggestions, but they respond to the "Yeah, but what if . . .?" questions that occur to the reader who is contemplating the sort of radical life changes that this program entails. Compulsive eating, however noxious it may be to those who suffer from it, represents a means of coping—however poorly—with life's problems. We need reassurance that we can replace this means of coping with something better, or we may be left unable to cope at all. Hirschmann and Munter provide this reassurance and offer an alternative to the diet mentality that takes such an enormous toll on our eating and our lives.

Janet Polivy, Ph.D.
C. Peter Herman, Ph.D.
University of Toronto

Acknowledgments

Our deepest appreciation to Karen Levine, whose skill, patient guidance, humor, and friendship made the writing of this book both possible and pleasurable.

Our heartfelt thanks to Richard A. Levy and Bert Wainer for their thoughtful attention to the manuscript and for their loving support.

Our gratitude to several others who read the manuscript and offered helpful comments—Frances Wells Burck, Alan Gelb, Jan Goodman, Laura Kleinerman, Carol Mager, Michelle Neumann, John Reilly, Judith R. Smith, Dr. Lucille Spira, Joan Stein, and to Linda Nagel for her assistance in developing the questionnaires.

Special thanks to our agent, Ellen Levine, for her skill, her support, and her tenacity, and to our editor, William Patrick, for his insistence that this book become the best it could be.

We would also like to acknowledge Martin S. Bergmann, Ernst and Gertrud Hirschmann, Janice La Rouche, Dr. Ruth Lax, Naomi Munter and the late Harold Munter, and Annemarie Rosenthal, from whom we have received so much. Our thanks also to Susan Gillespie, who kept home and hearth going, and to the children—Kate, Nell, Leta, Noah, and Nathaniel—for the many welcome (and sometimes not so welcome) interruptions in our workdays.

Introduction

If you count yourself among the people who feel compelled to eat even though you're not at all hungry, this book is for you. It offers a radical alternative to chronic dieting, a way to go beyond controlling your compulsive desire for food and start curing it.

"Control" means eating foods prescribed by others, according to their rules—what you do when you go on a diet. "Cure" means no longer needing rules and food restrictions, challenging many of your most deeply held convictions and dealing with something much more basic. Cure involves making peace with food, making peace with yourself, and returning to the weight that is appropriate for you. Cure is what this book is about.

You may be the sort of person who turns on the TV, remembers the pie in the kitchen, and polishes it off before the program's over, just because "it's there." Or perhaps you're the type who wants the pie, thinks about it all evening, but doesn't eat it. In either case, you feel that you live in a "thin or die" world and you're desperate. So first you diet and then you binge, despite the fact that study after study has proved that diets do not work and that the yo-yo effect of the diet/binge cycle serves only to make further weight gain inevitable.

We know that you, as a compulsive eater or chronic dieter, regard food as your problem. You believe that you must learn to curb your desire for food and eat less. As therapists who have worked with compulsive eaters for eighteen years, we've discovered that food is not really the problem at all. Food is delicious and nourishing, and no one should ever feel deprived of the enjoyment it offers. Your problem is that, as a compulsive eater, you consciously or unconsciously use food to manage your anxiety, to calm yourself when you feel stressed, and to bring comfort when you feel lonely or sad or afraid.

Because you alternate between using food to keep yourself comfortable and desperately trying to limit your intake, you've forgotten the true purpose of eating. For you, food no longer has anything to do with physiological hunger. Indeed, most compulsive eaters are rarely aware of when they are physiologically hungry. The signals that trigger your eating come from everywhere except your stomach.

Our cure for compulsive eating and overweight involves putting food back where it belongs. We are going to teach you to "legalize" food, to learn about yourself from your desire for food, and ultimately to eat your way out of your eating problem. We are going to show you how to lose weight by relearning how to eat. By the end of this process you will know how to feed yourself on demand—when, what, and how much you need.

Demand feeding opens the door to the fundamental cure for your addiction to food—the feeling of having been fed. You will discover that the simple act of feeding yourself when you're hungry has great psychological consequence. Our clients often report that feeding themselves on demand makes them feel stronger and generally less anxious. Many say that following our recommended way of eating increases their sense of entitlement and leads them to "feed themselves" in other ways as well.

We have discovered in our work as therapists and teachers that once you feel fed, you are in a position to tackle the emotional concerns that led you to misuse food in the first place. Once you feel fed, you'll have the awareness and the energy you need to deal with underlying problems that were masked by your "problem" with food.

Our approach to curing compulsive eating will enable you to

- give up dieting forever and discover that you eat much less without the restraints of a diet.
- learn to eat from physiological hunger and, perhaps for the first time, enjoy the enormous satisfaction of meeting that hunger with the foods you most desire.
- stop overeating and lose the weight that has been its by-product.
- move beyond your negative preoccupation with eating and weight into a fuller life.

If you are a chronic dieter, these goals may seem unattainable to you, and your skepticism is understandable. You are, after all, part of a terribly exploited group. A $20 billion diet industry thrives on your failure. You have been offered umpteen promises of cure, none of which have worked, and now we're saying that you can expect more than you've ever dreamed possible, that you can end your overeating and your overweight by doing away with all restrictions and eating freely.

We know from long experience that our suggestion that you give up food restrictions may trigger terror and incredulity. Compulsive eaters almost always believe that if they abandon diets and controls they will never stop eating. That is simply not the case, but we don't expect you to take our word for it. You will have to evaluate our arguments and the evidence presented in this book carefully and critically. And you will need a considerable amount of resolve to try something as new and different as what we offer. We think you will find our analysis compelling and that your fears will dissipate when you begin to take some steps that can change your life.

Over the years we have worked with perhaps eight hundred clients, one on one or in small groups, and as teachers and lecturers we have dealt with literally thousands more. We are therapists, not statisticians, and we have never been in a position to conduct the rigorous, double-blind studies that allow scientists to declare that something has been "proved." Nonetheless, our long experience with clients indicates that although 25 percent of people may feel frightened about such a radical change and give up on the program before it yields the desired results, the remaining 75 percent have a remarkable experience. They resolve their compulsive eating and in so doing change their lives. The examples throughout this book are drawn from our experiences working with people very much like you.

If you will stop yelling at yourself about your eating habits and your weight, if you will promise yourself—and truly mean it—that you will never diet again, we guarantee that, with our method, you will stop binging and gaining weight. Many of you will go on to become skillful, attuned "demand feeders" and return to your natural, lower weight. Even more important, you will develop a radically different feeling about yourself and your life.

One word of caution: although you may be tempted to follow some of our recommendations and omit those that most intimidate you, breaking an addiction to food is not something you can do successfully with a halfway approach.

Those who can take courage in hand experience the greatest success in the shortest period of time.

- Imagine being able to go to the cupboard and discover that most of the cookies in a box you opened several days ago are still there.
- Imagine having a terrible week, in which everything goes wrong and you feel depressed, yet not thinking about food except when you're hungry.
- And imagine not being on a diet, yet eating less and putting a stop to gaining weight. Not only does your weight stay the same without your "watching," but you can see how you'll actually lose weight once you get the hang of feeding yourself "from the inside."

We would be remiss if we didn't tell you that these ideas developed initially from our own problems with compulsive eating. In 1970, Carol Munter, determined to come up with an alternative to dieting, started a group for compulsive eaters, a group formed in the context of the developing women's movement. Susie Orbach, the author of *Fat Is a Feminist Issue,* was a member of this group. Many of you have probably read or heard about the radically new approach begun there and elaborated in her books. Several books were subsequently written about the need for women to examine their oppressive relationship to food and to their bodies. Kim Chernin, Geneen Roth, Nancy Roberts, Marion Bilich, and Carol Bloom are among the leading contributors to these developing ideas.

In 1982, Jane R. Hirschmann and Lela Zaphiropoulos took these ideas one step further. They developed a comprehensive approach to the feeding of children from birth through adolescence, an approach designed to remedy existing eating difficulties as well as to prevent children from developing food and weight problems. Their ideas are presented in the book, *Are You Hungry?*

Overcoming Overeating is the culmination of the work that was begun in 1970, which we have both expanded through the years. It further develops our unorthodox view of compulsive eating and combines it with an in-depth, psychological understanding of the underlying dynamics. We offer men and women a practical, step-by-step guide to the resolution of compulsive-eating problems.

We present this material here much as we do when we teach it. We argue for a new view of compulsive eating, then lay out the systematic approach that flows from our ideas. Our goal for each of you is the same as it is for all the people with whom we work. We believe that it is possible for you to break your addictive relationship with food and be free to live life unencumbered by an "eating problem." The proof of the pudding is in the eating!

– 1 –

Curing Compulsive Eating

The Compulsive Eater Identified

Picture this. You're walking down the street. You think you feel okay. You ate something a short time ago, but suddenly you start thinking about cookies and where the next bakery is. Or you're sitting, reading, not the least bit hungry, and you find yourself suddenly moving toward the refrigerator to get something to eat. Or you go out to dinner, have a fine time, stay nicely within the confines of your diet and come home feeling satisfied, but before you know it, you've polished off a cake direct from the freezer. After each of these episodes, you chastise yourself for eating and end up "feeling fat."

In each of these examples, your hand reached for food when you were not the least bit hungry. If you think about it nonjudgmentally, this behavior simply doesn't make much sense. Whether it's good or bad, it's certainly peculiar. Why eat if you're not hungry? Food's basic purpose, after all, is to satisfy physiological hunger.

Unfortunately, most of us have lost the capacity to regard our reach for food with any degree of objectivity. Even though the purpose of food is to supply our bodies with fuel, millions of people feel driven to eat, even when they are not at all hungry, and they accept this urge as a "bad" part of themselves that they will always have to keep in check. They expect to "watch" what they eat forever. They never question why so natural a phenomenon as eating should require such strict surveillance and control.

If your hand—or your mind—moves toward food when you're not at all hungry, you are, by our definition, a compulsive eater. You are compelled to think about food or how your body looks in situations where such thoughts have no logical place. We use the word *compelled* because we know that you have no control over these thoughts. They simply crop up in your mind. You suddenly get the urge to eat something while you're standing on the street talking to a friend. Or at a meeting you notice that you've lost the line of the conversation. Your colleagues are going through the agenda, but you're absorbed by painful, negative thoughts about the size of your stomach.

If you're a compulsive eater, you spend your days fighting your desire to eat. Some days you give in to your desire, and scream at yourself for your lack of willpower. Other days you resist the desire and feel virtuous and worthy of praise. On any given day, however, much of your mental life and energy is absorbed by thoughts about your eating, your weight, and your plans to control both. You've probably thought about these topics continually for many years. It may appear to others that you are leading a humdrum, average life, but they don't see beyond the surface of your daily activities. Despite appearances, you know that you are constantly preoccupied by painful thoughts about your body and eating. These thoughts envelop you, because compulsive eating is much more than an activity—it is an all-absorbing state of mind.

Some of you may regard yourselves as compulsive eaters; others may not. Some of you may think that compulsive eaters are fat, out of control, hard-core food addicts with deep-seated emotional problems. The truth is that compulsive eaters—men and women alike—come in all shapes and sizes and lead all kinds of emotional lives. What they share is their obsession with food and weight. This dual preoccupation with food and body shape is the hallmark of compulsive eating. Some compulsive eaters submit to their need for food and eat. Others control their desire for food and diet. In either case, the addiction to food rules the life of the compulsive eater.

In recent years, your private preoccupation with food and body image has gained cultural acceptance. It is considered chic, not problematic, to control your food comsumption and to work out until it "burns." Testimony to this fact is that at any given moment in this country, 80 million adults are dieting, that is, trying to control their desire for food. This culturally sanctioned fat phobia may have obscured your personal problem as a compulsive eater. Yet dieting, as we will demonstrate in the next chapter, actually creates and exacerbates compulsive eating and weight problems. Indeed, dieting has turned most of us into food junkies.

Look around the next time you're eating with friends. Has anyone who has finished eating left food on the plate? That is the sign of a noncompulsive eater, a rare bird in today's world. The food on his plate is there because he knows when he's had enough. It's true that sometimes he eats "too much," and sometimes he eats something simply because it looks good. However, most of the time he eats because his body prompts him to do so. He eats, in other words, because he's hungry. He likes food, but he's not hooked on it. Our intention in this book is to help you get unhooked. Phrases like "I'm hungry" and "I've had enough," which are alien to you now, can become a natural and effortless part of your vocabulary.

Physical Appearance: Compulsive eaters, who, as we've said, come in all shapes and sizes, are not necessarily fat nor are all fat people compulsive eaters. Much as we are accustomed to equating fat with gluttony, current research indicates that the shape of one's body is not necessarily a reliable indicator of one's relationship to food.

Fatness and thinness, according to this research, are complicated by many factors, primarily genetics. Some of you are genetically programmed to be large. For you, weight has no more to do with eating than does height. Tragically, you have probably been humiliated into regarding your large body as unnatural or believing that your size is the result of "greed" or "lack of willpower." If this sort of humiliation has brought you to the diet/binge cycle, you are probably even larger than you were "designed" to be.

Others of you may be compulsive eaters whose driven need for food is not reflected in your size. You have remained thin because your metabolism is such that either you don't gain or your binge and control cycles simply even out. We often hear from "thin" people who attend our workshops, "No one believes me when I say I have an eating problem. I struggle with food every day of my life. I know that I look as if I don't, but I'm obsessed with my weight." Hilde Bruch, author of *Eating Disorders,* calls such compulsive eaters "thin fat people."

Most of you, however, are compulsive eaters whose driven need for food shows. You weigh in above your natural weight because you overeat—you eat more food than your body requires. You reach for food when you are not physiologically hungry, and if you start out hungry, you continue to eat past the point of physiological satiation.

We define *overweight* as that weight which reflects the fact that you eat in excess of your body's needs. Notice that our concept of overweight bears no relation to the statistical concept of overweight reflected in height/bone structure/weight charts. These charts delineate statistical averages and have nothing to do with whether your body size is a reflection of overeating. We define normal weight as the natural weight you will return to once you cure your compulsive overeating.

No one can diagnose compulsive eating on the basis of size. Only you know if you feel compelled to eat or to control your eating. Only you know if you are a compulsive eater.

Self-Portrait: Compulsive eaters share not only their compelling need for food, but a view of their problem as well. All compulsive eaters consider themselves lacking in discipline and willpower—self-indulgent, greedy, infantile, out of control, weak, disgusting, and most important, *fat.*

Fat, skinny, or in between, all compulsive eaters *feel fat.* When they say that they "feel fat," they are really saying that they are "bad." Use of the word *fat* to mean "bad" is more significant as a sign of our culture's fat phobia than it is a description of body size. *Fat* in our society is an epithet.

Compulsive eaters consider themselves fat or bad because they measure themselves against two unquestioned cultural ideals and find themselves lacking. First, they accept the idea that there is an "ideal" body and that theirs is far from it; second, they believe that eating is something which must be "controlled." We will explore these and other cultural beliefs in Chapter 3. It is important to recognize, however, that your view of yourself as a compulsive eater is in perfect accord with the culture's views about bodies and eating. When you look at your body with disgust, chastise yourself for eating, and tell yourself that it's reprehensible to feel driven toward food, the culture nods agreement.

This society is not interested in why millions of people feel hooked on food. People are pressured to get rid of any evidence of their driven need for food, namely, to control themselves and lose weight.

Compulsive eaters consult us because they have "failed" to achieve these culturally imposed goals. They have gone on and off diets hundreds of times. "I'm beside myself" are the words we hear again and again. "I've been on every diet program imaginable and I've lost hundreds of pounds in the course of my life. I feel completely trapped. If I decide to diet in the morning, by dinnertime I'm on a rampage. I feel so hopeless."

The Compulsive Eater—A New Perspective

We see you, the compulsive eater, very differently from the way you see yourself. In our view, you have not failed. Rather, the solutions you have been offered, which are based on misconceptions of the nature of compulsive eating, have failed you.

Although you see yourself as weak-willed, self-indulgent, and lacking in self-discipline, nothing could be further from the truth. No one has ever tried more diligently to solve a problem than the chronic dieter. You have followed every recommendation ever made to you regarding how best to approach what you see as your problem. You have dieted and deprived yourself of food in endless ways. You have tried doctors, therapists, groups, hypnosis, exercise, meditation, chains on the refrigerator, retraining, fasting, et al. You have never spared energy, time, expense, or effort in your search for an answer.

Unfortunately, the answers you have found have been based on the idea that either you needed to develop better control over your eating behavior or abandon your own control to the rules of a diet. Indeed, you have been taught to condemn and restrain your eating when, in reality, weight control is not even the right problem to address.

The Problem of Control: It's no wonder that as a compulsive eater you feel hopeless. The way you've been told to deal with your problem—through control—puts you face to face with an impossible dilemma. You have been told *not to do* exactly what *you need to do*. If you're a compulsive eater, you are *compelled* to turn to food when you're in trouble. No amount of control, no amount of retraining or relearning "good" eating habits, will modify your need to eat.

Compulsive eating, like all human behavior, has meaning and significance. When you try to control a behavior like eating, you are simply commanding it to stop. You are saying, "It's bad. Don't do it," rather than doing something about the reasons underlying your compulsion. Diets say "don't eat," and as a result, they never work. They never address your need to turn to food.

Many people tell us, "I thought I had the problem licked. I lost a lot of weight last year and thought for sure that this time I'd be able to keep it off. Several months ago I started eating again and now I've gained back everything I lost."

You call it a failure when you are unable to stay within the confines of a diet. We call your failure to stay on a diet a "fight-back" response. When people are told to stop doing something they need to do, they don't simply stop. They fight back.

It is the thesis of this book that you do not have to spend the rest of your life trying to control your desire to eat. However, the cure for compulsive eating does require as a first step that you scrutinize your fight-back response to diets. In other words, you must take your reaching for food when you're not hungry—despite your best efforts to control yourself—as evidence that you have a deeper need which must be addressed.

Regardless of how it feels to you, we know that you are not being obstinate or self-destructive when you eat when you're not hungry. You eat at these moments because you must. If you thought about it, you'd probably say that in some "crazy" way, it feels to you as if food will "help." And you'd be right. For many years, compulsive eating has provided you with an important coping mechanism.

Self-Help: We believe that each time you reach for food when you're not hungry, you're trying to help yourself out of a difficult moment. In fact, the moment at which you eat may not seem all that difficult. All you know is that you want to eat.

We consider your need to eat at these moments a sign that something is making you anxious or uncomfortable. Each time you eat compulsively, you move from your unlabeled discomfort, to food then scold yourself for having eaten and for being too fat. This process of eating compulsively gets you off the track of what's really troubling you. And to make matters worse, you become convinced that the trouble is your eating and your weight.

Like every person, you, the compulsive eater, have unresolved emotional conflicts that cause anxiety. Your immediate problem, however, is the trouble you have grappling with your anxiety without the aid of food. You have a "calming" problem, not a food problem. Unfortunately, many of you have spent years desperately trying to solve the wrong problem. Controlling your eating and losing weight will never resolve your need to calm yourself with food.

Many compulsive eaters are aware that their eating is a symptom of other problems, and many of you probably have made a concerted effort to understand what drives you to eat. But recognizing the source of your anxiety does not help the fact that the only way you know how to cope with that anxiety is by eating. "I'm angry . . . I'm lonely . . . I'm depressed" are what you say as you desperately finish the pie. Even resolving your underlying conflicts will not necessarily put an end to your need to reach for food in order to calm down.

Nancy felt that she'd resolved a number of the difficult issues in her life. She'd left an unsatisfactory relationship, had recently been promoted at work, and was considering buying a house. She reported that she was feeling better about herself than she ever had. It was a mystery to her, then, why her weight continued to go up and down when she was feeling so much more secure.

It was only when Nancy began to feed herself in a new way that she saw why resolving her problems had not changed her eating. She realized that after years of dieting, she was completely disconnected from her natural need to eat. Nancy learned, as you will in the course of this book, that eating problems have to be solved in a unique way. Feeding yourself the way we will describe later goes beyond understanding and addresses the calming problems that give rise to overeating.

Compulsive eaters are a varied lot. They come with a variety of problems and with varying degrees of what might be considered mental health. Yet as dissimilar as they are, they have certain factors in common. First, they share a particular way of handling anxiety—they reach out for food. Second, they share the consequences of handling anxiety this way. After years of compulsive eating and chronic dieting, they have all disconnected the experience of eating from the experience of hunger. As we see it, the compulsive eater's lack of basic experience in getting hungry and feeling fed is at the heart of the problem. But therein lies the solution.

The Cure—The Hunger/Food Connection

We propose that compulsive eaters begin to cure themselves by repairing the damage their addiction to food has wrought; they must reconnect food and hunger. When compulsive eaters do this, it has a major impact on their calming problem, and as a result they have less need to use food for anxiety. When compulsive eaters break their addiction to food, they also lose weight. Here's how it works.

We are born knowing how to eat. We get hungry, we cry, and we are fed. Through endless sequences of getting hungry and being fed, we make contact with the world and learn that it meets our needs reliably. Early in life, feeding and calming are inextricably linked. Hungry infants panic, and when the world responds to their panic with food, they calm down. The feeding experience is at the center of myriad interactions and feelings that contribute to our sense of security.

Throughout life, feeding ourselves in response to hunger is both physically and psychologically nourishing. Noncompulsive eaters feed themselves when they're hungry several times each day. Each time they do, they are commemorating and reinforcing the good caretaking they experienced early in life. They are demonstrating to themselves, in this quite ordinary fashion, that they are attuned to their needs.

The situation of compulsive eaters is quite different. They do not have the daily experience of caring for themselves by eating when they're hungry. Their problem—using food to calm anxiety—has caused them to take food out of the original context of feeding. Their solution—dieting—has disconnected them still further from their natural need to eat. They use food as a symbol of the caretaking they once experienced as children in the hope that it will calm them as adults.

Compulsive eaters use food as a medication or salve rather

than as a fuel. They apply food to every possible problem except the one which food is designed to fix, namely, hunger. Food as a symbol of comfort is ineffective; it is not an antidote for anxiety. Food as a fuel in response to hunger, however, is most effective.

The cure for compulsive eating requires that you put food back where it belongs, a process we call "demand feeding for adults." You are going to go back to the beginning of your eating life and start over again, reestablishing the connection between food and hunger that was severed years ago.

The heart of our plan involves eating as often as possible in response to physiological hunger. The more often you eat when you're hungry—the more you become your own attuned caretaker—the less need you will have to resort to food when you're anxious. Ultimately, as the needs of your body begin to determine when, what, and how much you eat, you will reestablish your natural weight.

It is important to understand, however, the great significance of teaching yourself to eat differently. Feeding yourself on demand addresses the heart of your calming problem. It is the simplest and most basic way to care for yourself. The more you do it, the more secure you'll feel. And as you feel more cared for, you will be better able to think about your troubles rather than eat about them.

Food on demand will by no means solve all your problems, nor will it eliminate your anxiety. That's not necessary. What you need is to be able to live with your anxiety and give your problems their proper names. Demand feeding will make it possible for you to break your addictive relationship to food and feel more prepared to address your real concerns.

Right now, you believe that you have a problem with food and a problem with your weight. When you finish reading this book, we expect that you will see yourself differently, as someone who turned to food when you were in trouble and then called your trouble "food." Our goal for you, as for the people we work with, is to help you move from an obsessive concern about eating and weight into the pleasures and pains of real life.

The Plan

Ours is a three-part plan to cure compulsive eating. Phase 1 is called "Freeing Yourself." In order to begin to eat differently, you must first declare yourself independent of the prevailing cultural attitudes about bodies and eating. There are a number of actions you can take that will help you assert your new, understanding view of yourself and your compulsive eating.

Phase 2 is called "Feeding Yourself." It explains how to find out when, what, and how much food your body requires. It delineates the difference between physiological and psychological hunger and teaches you how to move gradually in the direction of demand feeding.

Phase 3 is called "Finding Yourself." It describes the addictive circuit in depth. It demonstrates how to turn what you once regarded as a deficit into an asset: to use the signal of what we call "mouth hunger" as a way to understand your emotional life.

Our plan works, but it does so only if you've had it with dieting. Therefore, we will begin with a presentation of our understanding of diets and your entrenched resistance to giving them up.

– 2 –

The Diet/Binge Cycle

Every reader of this book is familiar with the diet/binge cycle, but the way you got into the cycle may vary. Perhaps as a child you were told that you were too fat and were put on diets. Perhaps as a teenager you were confused and frightened by your developing body and decided to try to change it. Perhaps as an adult you found yourself attempting to eat your way out of a crisis and went on a diet to stop yourself from gaining weight. Or perhaps at some point in your life you just wanted to "feel better" by losing a few pounds. You probably didn't think much about going on a diet. It's a commonplace thing to do.

Although diets may be de rigueur, they are not innocuous. A diet is a serious step, because what is little understood is that every diet is rooted in negative feelings about oneself— feelings that range from disapproval to dislike to disgust to contempt to self-hate. The diet, as we shall see, inspires the binge. The binge results in even greater negative feelings about oneself, and the cycle starts again.

Diet/binge/self-contempt. Diet/binge/self-contempt. The cycle can, and often does, last a lifetime.

* * *

All of you have been "successful" dieters who have managed to lose weight. Most of you, however, have also regained the weight you lost. Current research indicates that 98 percent of all successful dieters regain their weight plus some. Indeed, most dieters regain their weight with a vengeance in less time than it took them to lose it. In a word, after the deprivation of dieting, they binge.

Why do we inevitably fail at the task of long-term weight loss? All of us believe that our failure is a personal one, that we lack self-control and discipline. Our hands, after all, are the ones that move from cottage cheese to cookies. No matter how many times the solution—the diet—fails us, we continue to believe that *we* are at fault.

It makes no sense to assume that the 80 million people who are currently dieting are somehow deficient, that they lack the discipline to achieve something they care very much about achieving, particularly when many of them succeed in their pursuit of goals in other spheres of their lives. Clearly there must be something inherent in every diet that ensures its ultimate failure.

The Fight-Back Response

Dr. Janet Polivy and Dr. Peter Herman have done extensive research at the University of Toronto to demonstrate that the restraints of a diet lead to a binge, regardless of the personality, character, or starting weight of the dieter. Through years of clinical practice, we have concluded that dieters are like tightly wound springs—the more restrained their eating, the tighter the spring. Once a dieter goes off his or her diet, the spring releases. The tighter that spring has been wound, the more forceful is its release. The more restrictive the diet, the bigger the binge.

Every diet—regardless of how long its book has been on the best-seller list, regardless of whether it tells you to count calories or grams, regardless of whether it tells you to eat grapefruit or bean sprouts—represents a spring readying itself to release.

Dr. William Bennett and Joel Gurin point out in _The Dieter's Dilemma_ that the body reacts to dieting as if famine had set in. Each time you diet, your body's metabolism slows down in order to store fat. The more you diet, the slower your metabolism, and with each successive diet it becomes more difficult, if not impossible, to lose weight.

Most current research confirms the view that the ultimate result of food deprivation is an increase in stored fat. Dr. Kelley Brownell of the University of Pennsylvania found that yo-yo dieting increases the activity of an enzyme that promotes the storage of fat. Losing and regaining cycles demonstrably increase body fatness.

From an evolutionary point of view, the survival of our species may be directly related to our body's ability to store fat in times of plenty for use in times of famine. Anne Scott Beller discusses this in _Fat and Thin: A Natural History of Obesity._ She points out that, like the animals who gain weight in anticipation of hibernating for the winter, people in northern climates were originally heavier and larger than those in southern climates. Their lives depended on it.

This physiological tendency to resist deprivation by holding on to supplies has its psychological counterpart. We all admire people who fight against adversity, who manage to survive against all odds. We recognize in them a life force that struggles to hold on to what is good and pleasurable despite all obstacles.

Most people, when threatened with deprivation of any kind—including self-imposed food deprivation—will fight to preserve what they have. The compulsive eater consents to deprive himself of food—to diet—but he inevitably "cheats." He calls it cheating because he fails to see that breaking the diet is his attempt to preserve supplies. He does not view his binging as the same kind of struggle against deprivation that he'd be the first to admire in another context. As we see it, the fight to hold on to something important—food—is at the heart of the diet/binge cycle.

Diets create rather than cure compulsive eating. That they also make us fat is a difficult, but essential, conclusion for any compulsive eater to reach. The idea of abandoning diets fills us with fear and hopelessness. No chronic dieter could take such a step without being completely convinced that dieting harms rather than helps. To this end, let us examine the diet/binge cycle even further.

The Urge to Diet

What gives you the idea to diet? What triggers the urge to lose weight? The idea is literally in the air. Living in a nation obsessed with food and weight control, you can't escape it. You embark on the diet/binge cycle because you feel dissatisfied with your body or fear what will happen to you if you don't gain control over your eating.

The stories of three people who attended our workshops are fairly typical.

It was early January and Sarah had just been asked by her closest childhood friend, Elaine, to be maid of honor at her forthcoming June wedding. Sarah's mind began to race. What am I going to do? I've gained twenty pounds this year and I needed to lose twenty before that. I've never been so fat. I've got to do something. I can't stand the thought of walking down the aisle like this. Let's see. When did Elaine want to go look for my dress? Two months from now? If I lose three pounds a week for eight weeks I'll be down at least twenty pounds by that time. I guess for the first twenty pounds I can use that diet I was on last year, but I'll have to find something new to lose the next twenty by June. If I'm very strict about it—and if I can get myself to exercise—I should be able to do it.

Five years ago John began his own public relations firm. Since then he had established a reputation within the field. With all the clients he could handle, he found himself turning people away. Then an international public relations firm approached him with the suggestion that he join them. The merger, if it happened, would be enormously rewarding for John, monetarily and creatively. He agreed to meet with the firm's representatives in two weeks, to talk terms. Needless to say, John was anxious about the meeting. He passed a mirror on his way to the local pizza parlor and noticed that he'd developed quite a paunch. When the hell did that happen? he wondered. I look terrible. I really need to get back in shape. How could I have let myself go these past few months? I must be up at least twenty pounds again. I've got to look better. Well, I've done it before and I can do it again. Starting tomorrow I'm going to cut out lunches and start counting calories. Maybe I'll start jogging.

Alice had always taken pride in her appearance. She worked very hard at staying slim, watching every morsel she ate. When invited to a dinner party she'd "let herself go" for the evening, but the next day she would skip breakfast and lunch. She had always found it quite easy to "watch her weight." In fact, she said she enjoyed it. It's like brushing teeth. She gets up in the morning and quickly reviews her food intake of the day before. Like a calculator, she's able to adjust quickly for yesterday's sins by planning her eating for the new day. When she booked a week's vacation at Club Med she dieted and lost ten pounds in preparation. That gave her the leeway to really have a good time and eat whatever she wanted on her vacation. When she returned from her vacation and stepped on the bathroom scale, she discovered that somehow, over the course of her week in the sun, she had gained back her ten pounds plus three. Her jaw dropped when she looked at the scale. She was furious with herself and began trying on the clothing she had bought before her vacation. *I never should have let go on vacation,* she told herself. *If I don't keep close reins on my eating I'll be a blimp in no time. It'll take me weeks to get back to my normal size.*

Sarah, John, and Alice, who are typical of most of us, were convinced that their bodies were a problem. All of them wanted to solve the problem through a diet, but that solution stemmed from a strong sense of "yuck" and fear. As a result they were doomed to fail.

The Yucks: Unbelievable as it may seem, millions of us get up every morning, look in the mirror, and say "Yuck." This is most disquieting. Not only is it unsettling that so many of us find our bodies unattractive, but saying yuck has serious consequences. Self-reproach, which so many of us believe engenders change, inspires little more than a sense of defeat. The more unacceptable you feel, the less able you are to change.

Anyone who has spent time with children knows that positive reinforcement leads to change and that blame and accusation end in stubborn compliance or outright rebellion. "I never saw anyone clean up a room faster than you did last week" always works better than "Look at your room. You're a slob. Get in there and clean up that pig sty before you do another thing." Children are clearly more willing to push themselves when they feel loved and supported than when they feel frightened and threatened.

Adults are no different. We also need to feel good in order to change. When you feel good about yourself you're open to meeting new people and doing new things. When you feel yucky you're more likely to hole up in your apartment. When you're confident that your boss likes you and thinks well of you, you are likely to produce good work. When you feel demeaned by your "superiors" you're less willing to offer your opinion. This simple idea—having to feel good in order to change—is at the heart of our approach to compulsive eating.

The Diet

"No more lunch." "No more sweets." "No more than 1000 calories a day." "No more protein before noon."

At the heart of every diet is a resounding *"No more."* Dieters, as we said, progress from feeling bad to feeling that they should restrict their eating. The particular method by which they do it is not important. At any given time there are dozens of options: liquid protein, foods eaten in a particular sequence, high-fiber, low-fat, high-fat, low-protein, high-protein, low-carbohydrate, and on and on. Regardless of what diet you choose, however, you are opting to limit your food choices. You are, in a sense, relinquishing control over what you eat.

To be sure, many people welcome the rules and regulations of a diet. They like the structure. They feel relieved to have the decisions about when, what, and how much to eat taken out of their hands. They find it easier to say "I'm not allowed" than to struggle with their needs and desires. They also feel virtuous and worthy. After all, we live in a culture that applauds control.

On the surface the decision to restrict food makes a great deal of sense and seems like a healthful thing to do. Restricting food in response to a yucky feeling, however, is far from benign. When you restrict your food intake because you find yourself disgusting—or because you are terrified of the consequences of *not* restricting it—you are essentially punishing yourself. You are saying that you eat too much, that you are bad for doing so, and that you must be controlled. The diet is the punishment for your "out-of-control" behavior.

Once you understand that diets are punishments for bad behavior, you can understand why they fail. Eating—overeating, undereating, any eating—is not a crime, but when you confine yourself by dieting, you are sentencing yourself as if it were. You are not questioning why you eat or what you can do about it. You are simply saying "*Stop.*"

Diets are fundamentally confinements much like prisons, and dieters, like prisoners, do time for not looking right. Prisoners share a common fantasy—rebellion. Regardless of how willingly a dieter enters the confines of a diet, she becomes sullen after a while and begins to think about breaking out. Convicts dream about the proverbial cake cum file. Dieters do very well without the file—they just dream about the cake.

The Binge

In light of what we've learned so far, it makes sense for dieters to dream of breaking free from diets. After all, a diet does nothing to change your need to eat. All your diet does is attempt to keep you from eating. It's a control mechanism. Remember the analogy to the tightly coiled spring?

Let's return to Sarah, who dieted so she would look acceptable at her best friend's wedding.

Sarah's diet was an enormous success. She lost thirty pounds in time for the wedding. For months she followed a rigid plan of diet and exercise. She waited until the last moment to buy her gown because she wanted to be at her thinnest for the occasion. Sure enough, she found her fantasy dress—a sheath she would never have had the nerve to put on her "former" body. As the day of the wedding approached, Sarah began to feel anxious. She wasn't quite sure why, but she found herself feeling more and more hungry.

At the wedding Sarah was greeted with a barrage of compliments. "You look fabulous. I would barely have recognized you." "How did you do it?" And so on. She marched down the aisle and turned to watch Elaine make her entrance. Her eyes welled up. She was happy for Elaine, with whom she had spent endless hours talking about how much they wanted to start their own families. Elaine was on her way. Sarah was hungry.

At the reception, a waitress passed a tray of canapés. Sarah saw her favorite, caviar and egg, nestled among the others, crying, "Eat me. Eat me." She thought, God. I love those things. But I can't take a chance. I've worked too hard to lose this weight. She walked away, but the waitress seemed to be tracking her. Look, she told herself, her mouth literally watering as she fixed her gaze on the tray. What difference is it going to make if I indulge a little tonight? I've been so *good* for so long. I can be *bad* just this once.

And Sarah ate, not just one canapé but several. And the cake and cookies that followed. While she appeared to be conversing with people, her mind was riveted on the trays of food being passed. The more she ate, the more she thought about eating, and the more disgusted with herself she felt.

The next morning Sarah looked at herself, felt fat, and berated herself as she had done for so much of her life. She then spent weeks eating and blasting herself for it. Every morning she told herself she was back on the diet, but by lunchtime her resolve had faded. She would eventually drag herself into the next diet, but couldn't yet muster the energy to begin.

Like Sarah, all dieters assume that life will be better in a smaller size. Yet the endless nature of the diet/binge cycle is proof that diets don't live up to their reputation. Not only are they punishments for bad behavior, but they *never* deliver on their promises.

Sarah had a mixed reaction to all the "compliments" she got at the wedding. On one level she loved them, yet she was aware that they made her uncomfortable. It seemed like a lot of attention. And in the back of her head she was aware that the compliments implied criticism of her former state. "You look so good I barely recognized you" is simply another way of saying, "You looked awful before." After hearing those "compliments" all evening Sarah went home, where she felt very much alone. Her loneliness made her sad and angry. Here she was, thin, but burdened by the weight of her feelings. Sarah, in response to those feelings, did the only thing she knew how to do—she began to eat. Her diet had in no way addressed her need to turn to food when she was upset; it had simply restrained her.

Every "successful" dieter discovers that after the initial exhilaration of "fitting in," life is every bit as problematic when you're thin. That discovery combined with the deprivation of the diet is additional fuel for the binge that puts you right back on the merry-go-round.

* * *

The first step toward curing your compulsive eating is to acknowledge once and for all that diets do not work. Whether you stick to a diet for one hour, one day, one week, one month, or one year, you will inevitably break out of its restraints. Yet no matter how many times you've gone off diets, not starting a new one seems next to impossible. Compulsive eaters can't imagine life outside of a diet without envisioning themselves eating everything in sight.

Reasonable people who have spent the better part of their adult lives riding the carousel of the diet/binge cycle are the first to acknowledge its limitations. "Sure," they seem to say, "it's true that I get on the horse and off the horse in the very same place." Then they pause and add, "But one of these days I'll grab the ring, and then everything will be different!"

Our hope that the next diet will end differently is a desperate one. We cling to the belief that diets can work because they seem like our ticket to a better life. They are also the only way compulsive eaters know to live.

– 3 –

Signing Up for a New Life

One More Time

The word is out. The mass media are filled with the news that diets don't work. Each talk show host announces the dismal failure rate of diets, yet at the end of the program concludes that we should not lose hope, we should just try harder! An astonishing conclusion. "Try harder" at what? If diets don't work, why should we try harder to stay on them? Time and again, we pick up the challenge, tuck away the confusing message about diets not working, and soon find ourselves enticed into yet another.

You know the scenario. You are standing in the checkout line in the supermarket. The magazine covers beckon: "A New You for Summer," "Thinking Your Way to Thinness," "A Firmer You in Ten Minutes a Day." Or you meet an old friend who has lost a lot of weight. She looks terrific. Your envy overcomes whatever inhibitions you might have about asking her how she did it. Or you jump on the wagon when a new diet plan hits the best-seller list.

All of us who hear the message that diets don't work resist it. We cling to the belief that *we* can find a way to make one work. This time will be different, we tell ourselves, and with that promise, we reenter the diet/binge cycle—one more time.

*   *   *

One would think that people who have spent a lifetime failing at diets would be relieved to discover that they no longer need to shoulder the responsibility for their failure to lose weight. But one would be wrong. We're not at all relieved—we're very upset. We want to keep dieting, and any diet that promises to make us thin for the summer is worth a shot. We know that by the time winter rolls around we'll be ready for our winter diet, but in the meantime, thin for summer is better than not thin at all.

What is so alluring about being thin for summer—or winter or spring or fall? What, beyond having visible pelvic bones, do we hope to achieve by getting thinner? Clearly, we believe that being thin will bring us something. How could we not? We are surrounded by that message and we buy it. Thin is definitely in.

We live in a society in which physical appearance and self-worth are equated. Bodies are used as symbols to sell every product imaginable, and all of us who have gone on diets are secretly hoping for a great deal more than a slimmer body. We are hoping for what that thin body symbolizes, which—as we will discuss—can be anything from general happiness to career success to a great sex life or a fancy new car.

The diet—the prescribed path to thinness—is our hope for a better body and a better life. Dieters, in their addiction to false hope, are very much like gamblers. A gambler who is told that the slot machines are rigged, that he can't win, does a surprising thing—he puts another quarter in the slot and tries again. If you ask him why he keeps playing he'll reply,

"It's the only game in town." Playing the slot machine, or any game of chance, is the way a gambler gives himself hope. Each time he pulls the lever on the side of the machine he thinks his ship will come in. Exhilarated as he watches the fruit spin before his eyes, he's crushed when he loses. But not for long. He'll play again, "one more time," to experience the elation of a possible win.

Diets are a game of chance that dieters play in order to maintain hope for a better life—in a thin body. To the compulsive eater the diet is the only game in town. Game? We use the word cautiously and in the most ironic sense. This is a game in which the quality of people's lives is at stake. Chronic dieters are trapped in the diet/binge cycle and can't see beyond it. Their worlds have become narrow, focused on pounds lost and pounds regained. This painful preoccupation keeps them from truly living.

Change Your Shape and Change Your Life

Our name for the diet game is "Change Your Shape and Change Your Life." It's a game that many people who feel bad about themselves play in the hope that they will feel better. This game is certainly well publicized, highly touted, and extraordinarily enticing, beckoning to us from billboards, from the pages of magazines, from TV, and from trusted family friends and physicians. It not only beckons, it demands our participation. The message is crystal clear—if you lose weight, you will have a happier, healthier, all-around better life.

In our culture, dieting, and the weight loss that presumably follows, is advanced as a great cure-all. If you feel sluggish, a diet will give you pep. If you feel isolated, a diet will make it possible for you to have new friends. If you feel unloved, a diet will bring you romance. Whatever the problem, be it physical or emotional, there is some diet that promises to cure it.

The moment we become embroiled in a hot game of Change Your Shape and Change Your Life, we are hard put to recognize what about our lives, other than our shape, needs changing. Painful as it is, we suffer this game for what it gives us—the hope that we may someday gain control over our lives, which is the motivating force behind Change Your Shape and Change Your Life.

The Motivation to Play: People in today's world have very little control over many important things in their lives. Satisfying jobs are scarce; nuclear disaster looms large; inflation escalates; hard-to-find housing is harder to afford; education and medical costs are overwhelming; drugs are alluring; love relationships don't often work out; and families fall apart. Most of us are overwhelmed by the plethora of problems that touch our lives, directly and indirectly.

Historically, when people have felt the least control over their lives they have turned to the realm of magic for support, and we, enlightened though we may be, are no different. As social crises deepen, magical and fad solutions to our problems become more and more popular.

On good days we try to think things through realistically. We develop a plan to find a job or an apartment. We join political organizations that promote our wish for a safer environment. We go with our spouse to a marriage counselor.

But not every day is a good day, and on those not-so-good ones we find ourselves wishing for a magical solution to our problems. Winning the lottery is one such solution. We know our chances are slim, but we enter the fantasy, particularly on a day when someone else wins several million. We imagine ourselves in their shoes. What would we do first?

Buy a big house or an apartment with a great view; the marriage would thrive in the right space. And then? A retirement income for the folks. And then? A vacation—three months around the world, first class. And then? Well, there would be contributions to the hungry. And on and on. We're elated, but before we know it, time has passed and we're dumped, abruptly, back into our narrowly budgeted lives. We all know that the lottery is a long shot, yet when we feel least able to control our lives, a long shot seems better than none at all.

Diets provide the same kinds of fantasies for people who feel out of control as do lotteries. And those fantasies are every bit as difficult to give up as that of hitting the right lottery number. You get in the shower. Maybe you've just had an argument with your kid; maybe you feel foolish about what you said on your date last night; maybe you're not thinking about much of anything, but you look at your body and feel disturbed. You start thinking about trying to do something about your weight. If you're an old dieting pro, you start making some calculations: If I start today, I'll lose five pounds this week, two each of the next, so in six weeks that'll be . . . , and you lose yourself in a reverie that feels good. And as long as you can stay lost in the fantasy you feel transformed! You've forgotten about the kid, the faux pas, the cellulite, the paunch. You're off to a new life.

Players in the game do not want to believe the evidence that the diet, their most accessible hope for transformation, does not work for them any more than the gambler wants to admit that the odds are against him.

Let's meet the players.

The Players: Think about the last twenty-four hours of your life. Try to remember getting out of bed, showering, dressing, eating, arriving at work, coffee break, working, coming home, going out for the evening. If you're a player in a game of Change Your Shape and Change Your Life, your day, as you reflect on it, was marred by unpleasant thoughts about eating, weight, and the shape of your body. The familiar litany haunts you: Yuck. Disgusting. I can't stand it. I have nothing to wear. My thighs keep rubbing together. I can't go out like this. I must do something about myself. I'm gaining again. I can't stop eating. It's been a week since I last exercised. My shirt buttons keep popping open. My pants feel so tight.

If you find it impossible to escape thoughts like these, you are probably much involved in the game. A genuine player has an endless supply of painful self-criticism directed toward her body, which, in a word, is *wrong*, in desperate need of fixing. She believes, in her heart of hearts, that if she were worthwhile she would be able to control it and berates herself cruelly for her lack of willpower.

The Rules: The rules of Change Your Shape and Change Your Life are simple. Each of the five basic rules represents a cultural idea, which master players never question.

First, you must agree that fat is bad. Second, you must believe that fat people eat too much. Third, you must accept that thin is beautiful. Fourth, you must assume that eating requires control. And finally, you must be convinced that criticism leads to change.

Let's begin.

Rule No. 1 — FAT IS BAD

No serious player at Change Your Shape and Change Your Life ever questions the assumption that fat is bad, because we live in a culture in which fat is no longer a description but has become an epithet. Fat people are regarded not simply as large but as unhealthy, unstable, unhappy, untrustworthy, unclean, and sadly, unlovable.

"The notion that body fat is a toxic substance is now firmly a part of folk wisdom," Dr. William Bennett and Joel Gurin write in *The Dieter's Dilemma*. They cite study after study that disproves any correlation between fat and most of the illnesses it is reputed to cause and conclude, "It is far easier to say fat is bad for you than to say I don't like the way you look." Several of the studies reported in that book indicate that some weight above the "norm" may even be beneficial.

Indeed, people in our culture go far beyond not liking the way fat looks. We internalize the notion that fat is bad at a very early age. One study by Sue P. Dyrenforth, D. B. Freeman, and Susan C. Wooley reported in "A Woman's Body in a Man's World" (from *A Woman's Conflict: The Special Relationship between Women and Food*, Jane Rachel Kaplan, ed. Prentice-Hall, 1980) presented a group of toddlers with line drawings of children who varied by weight, race, and sex. Each child was asked to point to the child "you especially like," the child "you don't like very much," "someone who is weak," "someone who is happy a lot," and so forth. Every group of preschoolers preferred the line drawings of thin children and associated the drawings of fatter children with negative traits.

Once these children reach school age their attitude about fat is already well ingrained. A number of studies reported in the same article have found that schoolchildren describe children with round, fleshy body types in a pejorative way, using words like *lazy, mean,* and *dirty.* The *Wall Street Journal* for February 11, 1986, reported a random sample of fourth-graders in which 80 percent of the girls were already on diets, attempting to escape negative stereotyping. This staggering statistic demonstrates how early the pressure to conform begins. What a tragedy that nine-year-olds are caught up in Change Your Shape and Change Your Life. It takes a great deal of courage to withstand the pressure of this society's values and mores. Fourth-graders certainly can't do it. Even adults find it almost impossible.

Adults in this society cling to the belief that fat is bad with a fervor bordering on the religious. The modern American's censorious views of fat and eating are comparable to the Victorians' views of sexual desire in women. The Victorians were advised to summon their self-control when it came to sexual feelings; we are advised to summon our self-control when it comes to eating. The Victorians were warned that sexual desire would lead to physical and psychological illness; we are warned that any weight above the norm will result in physical and psychological illness. The Victorian bound herself in a whalebone corset; fat people today have their jaws wired shut, their stomachs stapled, and their thighs pared down.

Committed players at Change Your Shape and Change Your Life go to extraordinary lengths to win—to rid themselves of "evil." Restraint is a beginning, self-deprivation the next step. And to finish the game? We are offered surgery.

Rule No. 2 — FAT PEOPLE EAT TOO MUCH

Any experienced player at Change Your Shape and Change Your Life will tell you that the reason people are fat is simple—they eat too much. "Look at that fat person eating the ice cream," a player says. "How can he do that!"

What this player neglects to notice is that sitting next to the fat person eating ice cream is a thin person eating a banana split. Susan and Wayne Wooley, psychologists at the University of Cincinnati College of Medicine, cite many studies in an article for the *Journal of Applied Behavior* (12, 1979) which conclude that fat people eat *the same amount of food or less* than normal-weight people. In other words, fat people don't necessarily eat more dessert, or more anything, than thin people. And although they are loath to admit it, most players, at one point or another, have recognized this truth. Each of us has a cousin or a friend who is thin as a rail and packs food away as though there were no tomorrow. Some of us have even cried about how unfair it is. "She can eat half a chocolate cake and nothing shows. All I do is look at it and I gain five pounds, all in my thighs."

Given that fat and thin people have been documented as having similar eating habits, it's reasonable to ask why are some of us fat and others thin. The answer seems to be twofold.

People who are gaining weight are clearly suffering from an imbalance in the amount of food they ingest and the rate at which they burn that food for energy. We gain weight when we eat more food than we burn. The point at which any given body stops burning and starts storing fat, however, is specific to that body. Fat people may not eat more than thin people do, but they burn the same amount of food less efficiently. As Polivy and Herman point out in *Breaking the Diet Habit*, "Fat people do not need appreciably more calories to maintain their weight than do normal-weight people. There is a range of 'maintenance' calories required to maintain a stable weight for most people."

A skilled player at Change Your Shape and Change Your Life responds to this information by upping the game's ante. If fat people get fat by eating normally, then fat people simply have to eat less and less and less. Fat people, in other words, have to find out just how much, or little, food will turn them into thin people.

Short of starvation, such efforts are destined to fail. As explained in *The Dieter's Dilemma*, research indicates that each of us has a setpoint. Most adults are able to diet down to a weight below their setpoint or eat up to a weight above it, but when the diet/binge cycle is over the weight will return to the setpoint level. The setpoint is like a thermostat set to a certain weight. Any change in climate, and the setpoint brings the body back to its orginal setting.

People come in different shapes and sizes. Some of us are genetically programmed to be fatter than others in much the way that some are programmed to be taller than others. Although the message in our culture is that our bodies are endlessly elastic, the truth is that the shape of our bodies is programmed much like the length of our legs or the color of our eyes. When we tamper with our program, we get into trouble. As we have shown, diets wreak havoc with our program, leading to overeating and ultimately to overweight.

The truth that we can't all be the same shape is too painful for most game players to accept. It means that they will always live life feeling that their body is, in a word, *wrong*. Consequently, serious players try not to hear the news about genetics and metabolism. Their hope is to become thin, and they will not, under any circumstances, allow that hope to die.

Rule No. 3 — THIN IS BEAUTIFUL

If fat is bad, then thin is good, thinner is better, and thinnest is best. Immersed as we all are in a culture that worships the bare-bones model and the hard-edged corporate executive, we find it hard to recognize the extent to which these idealizations are simply passing fashions like bustles and spats. Yet ideals like thinness *are* historically determined. They express changes in circumstances and values.

When food was less plentiful, fat was symbolic of wealth. Wealthy people, after all, had enough food to eat in excess. Today, thinness is emblematic of having so much that one can choose to do without. In other words, if we weren't sure about our next meal, we probably wouldn't eat a cucumber for lunch. The rotundity of Queen Victoria was once symbolic of power and wealth and control. Those same attributes are now embodied by Nancy Reagan in considerably less flesh.

"Fine," says our player at Change Your Shape and Change Your Life, "I'll give you that. If I were living in Victorian England I wouldn't mind being fat. But I'm not living in Victorian England and I'd damn well rather be thin." It's extremely difficult for any of us to separate ourselves from our cultural standards. It's almost impossible to see that the body shapes we most admire reflect the taste of our times rather than an absolute aesthetic.

We all want to be in fashion. Unfortunately, we are not as elastic as fashion would have us. The fact that we come in a variety of shapes makes life particularly painful for those of us whose shape is not currently in vogue. Our pain is increased, however, because the body type of the moment represents qualities far beyond fashion.

Those of us who wake up each morning and say "too fat today" are expressing more than a wish to be "in with thin." We are, in effect, saying that we are unacceptable as we are and that we must better ourselves. We believe that if we could reshape our bodies to look the way "those people"— the ones who seem to have it all—look, we would then be better and more acceptable.

Historically, women have been most cruelly trapped by this dynamic. Having had little access to political and economic control, they could only try to reshape themselves to please those upon whom they were dependent. Not only have women tried to change the shape of their bodies, they have also tried to change every aspect of themselves—their faces, their hair color, their voices, their postures, and every nuance of their behavior. As Susie Orbach and Kim Chernin have explored in detail, no woman, in a culture that discriminates against her, can feel that her body is the right body.

Women exemplify all those who have been powerless. Powerless people do two things: they try to please those on whom they are dependent, and they attempt to be as much like those in power as possible. Sadly, the more they idealize people in power, the more they hate themselves.

Eighty percent of adult women, as reported in *Vogue* magazine, May 1986, feel they are too fat and want to make themselves thin. Why thin? The male of our species is, by nature, thinner, harder, and more muscular than the female, who is rounded and curved by fat deposits on breasts and hips. Why does a woman strive to be more like a man? Because despite the great inroads women have made, men continue to have more power and control.

This is not to say that men are not also players in the game of Change Your Shape and Change Your Life. Unrealistic standards for body size and shape—more muscle, firmer bodies, youthful, trim figures—now apply to men as well. It's no longer enough for a man to be good at what he does; he has to look the part as well. As men feel less powerful at the workplace, in the community, and at home, they become more subject to the lure of the game of body shaping.

Change Your Shape and Change Your Life is about power and control. All of us who play are attempting to recreate ourselves, to become someone we are not. As we strive endlessly to lose weight, to take up less space in the world in an effort to mimic those whom we perceive as powerful, we are engaged in a process of self-destruction. It is a cruel irony that in our efforts to get more—to make ourselves more powerful—we must make ourselves into less.

"You can never be too rich or too thin." Our young, anorectic girls embody the most tragic outgrowth of this belief. They represent the ultimate effort to be thin. As Susie Orbach demonstrates in *Hunger Strike*, these girls end up literally destroying themselves as they attempt to take charge by eradicating fat—their symbol of need, desire, and femininity.

Fortunately, most of us do not win the game of Change Your Shape and Change Your Life; but as players we don't perceive our failure as fortunate. Indeed, each time we fail to get as thin as we wish to be, we feel defeated, scold ourselves, and gird up for the next round.

Rule No. 4 — EATING REQUIRES CONTROL

Players in the game of Change Your Shape and Change Your Life strive constantly to achieve better control over their eating. Such control is at the very heart of the game. The topic pervades discussions among the players. They trade food plans, recipes, health spa information, and tips on the latest exercise regimen designed to alter metabolism. Players are world-class experts on the subject of control, a subject, we might add, that is of great importance to the society at large.

The control of eating begins early in the lives of all of us. Although there has been some debate over the years about the relative merits of demand versus scheduled feeding for infants, no one ever questions the necessity for control over eating. We discuss only when regulation should begin. Those infants who are fed on demand, whose cries of hunger determine the times at which they are fed, are taught soon after they can feed themselves that their eating must conform to the family rules about when, what, and how much to eat. Infants fed on a schedule learn earlier to conform to external regulation.

As a society, we regard eating in much the same way that

we regard the matters of toilet training and sex. We see eating as something that must be socialized through the use of external restraint. Not only is there a time and a place to eat, but some foods are forbidden and must be meted out sparingly. It is as if we believe that without eating rules, we would all be insatiable.

Players never question the idea that they must control their eating. If anyone were to suggest to them that if they stopped controlling what they ate, they would eat less, they'd consider the suggestion ridiculous and quite dangerous. Scheduled eating is an unquestioned part of the social order. In the minds of players, the workplace, the school, and the family require such regulation. For the sake of the social good, we, as individuals, must give up our right to determine when, what, and how much to eat.

Veteran players work to refine their control over eating. They no longer settle for simple regulations—three meals a day, appetizer before the entrée, dessert after the main course. They create elaborate, carefully timed menus that include various combinations of foods in specific order and in precise amounts. The more regulated they feel, the more relaxed players become.

Rule No. 5 — CRITICISM LEADS TO CHANGE

We said that diets are punishment for not looking right. Lest you have any question about this, consider some of the cruel techniques recommended to dieters. "Put a picture of yourself at your heaviest on the door of the fridge." "Wear something a little bit tight, a bit uncomfortable, so you'll be reminded to eat less." "Tell yourself that there will be no new clothing until you lose twenty pounds."

In other words, dieters are encouraged to dump on themselves in order to bring about the desired change in their body shape. Serious players at Change Your Shape and Change Your Life never question this approach. Painful as it is, they spend most of their unoccupied moments chastising themselves for their uncontrolled eating and their weight. They are convinced that if they tell themselves that they are bad, the self-reproach will lead to self-improvement.

Every dieter has learned that reproaches don't work. The result of walking around in tight clothing, for example, is feeling uncomfortable, and when compulsive eaters feel uncomfortable they *need* to eat. Eating, for them, is a way to feel better. After eating, they scold themselves, feel bad, and then have to eat again.

The truth is that people never scold themselves into significant change. Change, we repeat, comes about through nurturing support. It's hard for compulsive eaters to see this. It seems to them that if they feel bad enough, they'll be inspired to change.

This notion that running a race is best done by hitting yourself over the head at the starting line stems from a thoroughly wrongheaded, yet deeply cherished cultural belief. We have all been taught that you can do anything if you just put your mind to it. Pull yourself up by the bootstraps, nose to the grindstone—it's simply a matter of will.

Try and try again seems, at first, to be an extremely optimistic and encouraging idea, but it is the proverbial wolf in sheep's clothing. Curing compulsive eating requires much more than pulling yourself up by the bootstraps. Compulsive eating is a serious, very real problem that cannot be resolved through willpower. If willpower were the answer to compulsive eating, diets would work. Compulsive eaters have plenty of willpower. What they lack is self-esteem and the ability to calm themselves down. In fact, the self-loathing that motivates the game is precisely what exacerbates the problem of compulsive eating.

Most of us continue to play the game despite being repeatedly made aware of its failure to deliver. We play because we are desperate. We are struggling—in a hostile environment—to gain some control over our lives. Unfortunately, Change Your Shape and Change Your Life promises a kind of control we simply cannot have. It makes two promises, a new shape and a new life, and doesn't deliver on either one.

Although most compulsive eaters are aware of the diet's failure to deliver the real control they seek, most of them cannot imagine an alternative. Flawed as it is, they do see dieting as the only game in town. This is not surprising.

There is enormous social pressure to play and continue to play Change Your Shape and Change Your Life. The pressure is effective because we have each internalized the rules of the game so well.

When people say, "Oh, you've lost weight. How wonderful you look," we feel complimented. We agree that thin bodies are wonderful. When a friend summons up the courage to tell us that we appear to have gained weight and ought to do something about it, we feel ashamed at first, then agree. We perceive such criticism as being in our best interests. When people suggest a new diet, we're happy to try it. We like hearing about new ways to control ourselves. We feel that we are better when we eat with restraint. We live in a culture obsessed with control, and we admire discipline and abstinence.

* * *

To tell yourself and others that Change Your Shape and Change Your Life does not work and that you are no longer going to play requires great strength and courage. It means defying generally accepted cultural ideas that you formerly believed wholeheartedly. Not only must you bow out of a game that everyone considers essential to life, but you must do so without knowing what the results of your move will be, and you are understandably quite fearful about it. Painful as it is to play and lose and play and lose again, the game organizes the lives of its players, who are totally absorbed by it. They talk about it, think about it, and plan their days around when and what they are going to eat. Asking a chronic dieter to leave the game is like asking someone to leave an unhappy home. Home may be unpleasant or uncomfortable, but it's home nevertheless.

We have confidence, however, that compulsive eaters can leave home—the game—behind and go on to lead more satisfying lives. Our confidence is based on the perspective we have about you and your eating. We think that you are closer than you realize to saying "no more" to Change Your Shape and Change Your Life. We see you, the compulsive eater, as a rule breaker. As often as you've gone on diets, you've gone off them. We see you as someone fighting back against restrictions that exacerbate rather than help your compulsive eating problem.

– 4 –

Rethinking the Problem

The Rebellion of Eating

You, the compulsive eater, feel like a hopeless case. You have spent the better part of your life trying to change your shape—dieting, scolding yourself, taking laxatives, forcing yourself to throw up—and your efforts have consistently failed. You live in a fat-phobic society, doomed by what you regard as your lack of willpower.

We, however, don't see you as a hopeless case at all, and we don't regard your lack of willpower a lack. As we've said, we consider your eating in response to the restraints of a diet a fight-back response indicative of your strength of character. You resist even your own attempts to deprive yourself of what you need.

When we spoke earlier about diets we said that they were really a form of punishment for having an "unacceptable" shape. If you are fat or feel fat, you have absorbed the message that you are unacceptable and that if you lose weight you will become acceptable. You've spent years going through the motions of one diet or another in an apparent effort to look the way people say you should look, but you've never succeeded. One way to regard your inability to lose weight is to see it as your refusal to buckle under to discriminatory standards of acceptability.

From this perspective, your failure to lose your fat has been your way of saying, "I want to be accepted as I am." Every time you've gone on a diet to gain acceptability, you have binged and thereby said, "I will not submit to negative judgments." You have, in other words, stood your ground despite extreme social pressure to do otherwise. To be sure, you suffer from your excess weight and your addiction to food, but you have not changed your shape nor have you deprived yourself of food. Your unwillingness to do so represents your unwillingness, on one level, to accept the indictment of this culture. More important, it represents your insistence that you will continue to use food to calm yourself until you no longer need to do so.

Unfortunately, you, as a product of our culture, don't appreciate your stance for what it is. Our praise probably seems strange and untrustworthy to you. Despite your consistent refusal to give up food, you have not allowed yourself to feel at all good about who you are. Quite the reverse. At the very same time that you refuse to change yourself into an acceptable form, you look at yourself with self-reproach and self-loathing, call yourself names, and consider yourself a failure.

Your fat and eating symbolize your unwillingness on one level to accept a cultural indictment, which you have, on another level, internalized. You are caught in a bind in which you cannot possibly feel good about yourself.

It is upsetting, but understandable, that you continue to share the prevailing view that eating and fat are bad. It is remarkable, however, that you have had the strength to stand up to that viewpoint and continue eating. As a matter of fact, each time you break a diet with a binge, we see it as the healthy part of your saying "no more!" Every time you eat, you are resisting the contempt that underlies your efforts to control your eating and your weight. Contempt and re-striction foment resentment and rebellion. You are, in effect, a rebel with the healthy impulse to eat and soothe yourself as best you can when you feel troubled.

Beyond Rebellion

We understand that you don't see yourself as a rebel, but try the definition on for size. We think it fits. We think that bur-ied under your layers of self-contempt is not a thin person wanting release, but a rebel demanding to be heard and understood. You the hopeless case feel out of control and despondent because you've bought the line that you're a fail-ure at the idealized task of body shaping. But you the rebel are a success. You break the rules and assert your right to eat what you want and look as you do. The compulsive eater is, in an interesting way, a rebel in constant protest against what has, by now, become her own imposition of cultural standards and judgments.

Unfortunately, the effectiveness of your rebellion has been limited. Your continuous naysaying represents a reaction rather than real freedom. You are told to diet and lose weight. You do it for a while and then say "No, I will not live under these restrictions." Then the scenario repeats. In order to break into the cycle you will have to go beyond reacting, beyond saying no. Eventually you must find some-thing affirmative to replace your no. You will have to artic-ulate a better plan. A rebellion without a plan for the future is ineffective and leads to anarchy.

Before you can make a plan, however, you must get out from under your internalized contempt. Although the social pressure to look and eat a certain way is extreme, your own versions of these cultural dictates are far more cruel and in-sidious. You no longer need anyone to remind you that you are bad for not being thin and for using food the way you do. Your own voice is far more contemptuous than those which surround you.

You are probably not fully aware of all the ways in which you've internalized the cultural contempt for eating and flesh. Your rebellion against these attitudes has been unconscious. As you gradually become aware of how you treat and talk to yourself, it will be helpful to recognize three truths. First, that binging is a reasonable response to the restrictions of dieting. Second, that your unwillingness to give up food and buckle under to the pressures of our culture represents a rebellion rooted in self-respect. And third, that food has been a friend, a source of comfort to you, over the years.

When you stop condemning yourself for eating and, instead, start observing your behavior, you will discover a number of interesting elements about your reaching for food compulsively. We see your eating as an important effort on your part to help yourself.

The Linguistics of Eating

If you were to ask a compulsive eater at the moment he reaches for food "Why are you eating?" he'd respond, "I don't know. I just want it." If you were to ask "Are you hungry?" he'd probably find the question confusing. He wouldn't go quite so far as to actually say "What's hunger?" but he might as well. "I just want it," he would say. "I have to have it."

Indeed, for the compulsive eater, eating is rarely triggered by feelings of physiological hunger; instead, compulsive eaters eat when they feel discomfort. Most often, compulsive eaters do not know what, specifically, is causing their discomfort. They often do not get to the point of *experiencing* the discomfort that triggers their eating. What they do experience is a need to eat, and they invariably feel fat, that is, angry with themselves, after the moment of eating—the moment of peace—has passed.

The compulsive eater, as he or she moves from unlabeled discomfort to eating to self-contempt, is making a kind of translation. But instead of translating from English to French the way a linguist might, compulsive eaters translate feelings that make them uncomfortable into feelings of fat.

You are probably familiar with this process.

You find yourself at the refrigerator, not knowing why or how you got there; you only know that you have a strong urge to eat. You reach for food, and for a few moments it's you and the food. The world recedes. Once the eating is over—a few minutes, a few hours, or a few pounds later—the world returns and you are confronted with a different set of feelings and a different set of thoughts to accompany them, thoughts you've had again and again over the years. Why did I do that? How could I? What am I going to do about this weight? I've nothing to wear. Oh, I feel so awful. And on and on and on.

What happened? You weren't hungry, yet you felt like eating. You ate, and now there's a lot of ugly noise in your head. The discomfort, still unnamed, that triggered your eating in the first place, has not been alleviated, but its form has changed. Your initial feelings of discomfort have been replaced by a series of unpleasant thoughts about your eating, your lack of control, and the size of your body. You are now speaking to yourself harshly, with anger. These self-accusations are, perhaps, more uncomfortable than the original discomfort that sent you to food.

Whenever you eat compulsively, you are translating a nonspecified discomfort into a concern about eating and body size. If someone were to ask you after an eating episode what your problem was, you'd say it was your eating or your weight—and that's what you would believe—but such is not the case. Your real problem is your inability to sit with what-ever is troubling you and speak about it in its own language. Rather than face your problems and explore them, you eat. Once you have eaten, you make a translation from the language of feelings to the language of fat.

After you've eaten, you feel fat. You don't like feeling fat, but it has its advantages. First of all, it's a familiar old prob-lem, an erstwhile friend you may not like very much. Sec-ond, the problem of fat appears to be easily solved. As long as you regard your problem as one of fat, you can continue to believe that it can be dieted away. Let's look at some spe-cific examples of how this translation works.

Judy walked into work one day and discovered that the pro-motion she'd been hoping for had been given to someone else. She spent most of her morning in the ladies' room, fighting off her tears. In desperation, she asked her closest friend to meet her for lunch. She gobbled her food, then stopped at a bakery on her way back to the office. All after-noon she kept reaching into her desk drawer for cookies. She bought some premium ice cream on the way home and spent the evening binging. The next morning she felt fat and disgusting. Her binging continued for a few days until she finally roped herself into a diet. What happened? Judy had some feelings—disappointment, inadequacy, anger, envy, fear about her future—and unable to cope with them, she ran to food. As a result, Judy ended up focusing on the "problem" of her weight.

Ray and his wife were told that their bid for a house had been accepted, and they went out to celebrate. But Ray no-ticed that his celebration continued the next day and the day after that. As a matter of fact, it continued for much of the next month, and by the time of their closing he had regained all the weight he'd lost the previous summer. Why was Ray eating? We'll never really know. Whatever triggered it was eaten away. Possibly Ray felt elated—no one in his immediate family had ever owned a house. Possibly he felt uneasy with the notion of outstripping his family. Or possibly he had concerns about his new lifestyle. Would he be able to keep up with his payments? What if something happened to his job? Whatever Ray's concerns, his eating led to a catch-all-catch-nothing solution. Ray put himself on a strict diet.

Both Judy and Ray became preoccupied with feeling fat and out of control. They made a translation from feeling language to fat language.

1. An event disturbed their equilibrium.
2. They ate.
3. They felt fat and began to diet.

Compulsive eaters use feelings of fat as a catch-all category. Let's look at the examples. Judy initially felt disappointed and angry. Once she finished eating, she felt fat. We can speculate that Ray felt elated and frightened. Once he finished eating, he felt fat. Both Judy and Ray may very well be fat, by our current definition of fat, but the shape of their bodies is not their *real* problem, which is that they couldn't manage whatever they were feeling without going to food.

Food was the only way Judy and Ray knew to calm themselves. In that regard, perhaps the food worked for the moment, but once they finished eating, they were angry at themselves. When compulsive eaters get angry at themselves and call themselves fat, they are really saying that they should not have needed help and that there was something wrong with the feelings that led them to food in the first place.

Popular wisdom has it that people who are hooked on

food are set on destroying themselves. We believe quite the opposite, that each time compulsive eaters reach for food they are feeling uncomfortable, whether or not they know it, and are attempting to help themselves. We regard these efforts at self-help, regardless of their effectiveness, as life-saving devices deserving of great respect.

Food Feels Good and That Ain't Bad

You reach for food at a difficult moment in an attempt to help yourself. Is that a crime? Most people say your eating is self-destructive. We say that you eat when you are troubled, and that you are thereby trying to help yourself in the best way you know.

Your discomfort may stem from a feeling about your situation at that moment, from your general emotional state, from a thought you had seven thoughts ago, or from a nasty remark you made to yourself about your appearance when you glanced in the mirror. Indeed, if you have a difficult time feeling happy, your discomfort may even stem from feelings of eiation. Regardless of the source of your discomfort, you end up at the same place—the refrigerator door. Whenever a thought, feeling, or situation makes you uncomfortable—upsets your balance—you feel driven to eat.

* * *

When we reach for food compulsively, we are reaching back in time. As we've said, food, for all of us, represents one of our earliest experiences of being comforted. Even as adults, most of us feel cared for when someone takes the trouble to prepare a meal for us or treat us to one. All of us, in a primitive way, connect food and eating to our earliest experiences of being cared for and given pleasure. Consequently, food is a logical place for a compulsive eater in distress to turn.

The impulse to reach for caretaking when you feel needy

is a good one. But for adults, food remains only a symbol of nurturing. It soothes, but only in a symbolic and temporary sense.

Eating does not solve the complicated problems that trouble most adults. Judy's and Ray's feelings existed before they ate and will continue to exist after they eat. Although they get angry with themselves for eating, their turning to food is neither bad nor good. It's the way they calm themselves, if only for a moment.

Eating compulsively is like applying ice cream to a cut on your leg. When you reach for food, you are demonstrating that you know something about being taken care of and that you know enough to seek help. You care enough to want to comfort yourself. The food you reach for, however, does not have the properties to cure anything but physiological hunger.

Adults cannot effectively calm themselves by reaching back, which is essentially what we do when we attempt to soothe ourselves with food. We feel uncomfortable; we eat; we yell at ourselves; we swear to shape up and slim down; and then we feel relieved. Our relief, however, is evanescent. Dieting will not help either the source of our discomfort or the fact that when we feel uncomfortable we turn to food.

Instead, we have to be able to calm ourselves in the present, to think about what troubles us in the here and now, and to sit with our feelings of discomfort. Reaching for a symbol is not nearly as effective as taking care.

Eating Your Way Out of an Eating Problem

We want to give you, the rebel, a plan that will enable you to live your life without using food as a salve. As we see it, you have two problems. First are the troubles that trigger your eating. Second is your need to turn to food, rather than to your thoughts, for help.

Much as we'd like to, we cannot solve the many problems that send you to food. Fortunately, you don't have to solve those problems in order to stop your compulsive eating. In fact, we believe that things work the other way around. You have to begin with your eating, to get your food problem out of the way so that you can begin to clarify the real issues that trouble you.

How, if not through controls like diets, do you get food out of the way? Ironically, the way to do it and move on with your life involves eating. Ultimately, you will be able to recognize real hunger and eat in response to that hunger rather than in response to a generalized discomfort. You will be able to use food, which you've always identified as the problem, to transform yourself into someone who can look at problems and think them through. You will reharness the energy you put into worrying about food and weight and focus it, instead, on the issues that limit your life.

We are now going to present a step-by-step plan to help you end your compulsive eating. The first step is to assert a new and accepting view of your body and your eating. Phase 1 of our plan involves transforming your secret rebellion into open, affirmative action.

The Plan
Phase 1

Freeing Yourself

– 5 –

I Am What I Am

The If-Only Syndrome

Compulsive eaters live a life of "if only." "If only I could stop eating." "If only I could lose ten pounds." "If only I were thin." There is, of course, nothing wrong with wishing for a different and better life. There are problems, however, when compulsive eaters say "if only." The first is that "if only I were thin" is really another way of saying, "I hate myself the way I am." The second is that "if only" is a wish for magical transformation, not a realistic approach to change.

People rarely know how to say "I want to be different from the way I am" without putting themselves down at the same time. We've shown that when you put yourself down in an effort to change yourself, the healthier part of you refuses to budge. When you say "I'm disgusting, I have to lose weight," that healthier part of you heads for the fridge.

We understand that you want to be different from the way you are. We also know that, ironically, accepting yourself as you are is a prerequisite for changing.

Giving up the if-only syndrome makes it possible for you to begin to resolve your compulsive eating problem and to lose weight. Concretely, this means accepting your body in its current shape, living *as if* you will never lose another ounce. Understandably, this suggestion strikes panic in the hearts of those who live by the if-only syndrome. They feel that accepting the status quo means living a life of misery.

Although it may seem as if we are asking you to resign yourself to a life in a fat body, resignation is not what we're recommending. We are suggesting that you learn to live life whatever your weight. And we can reassure you that we see acceptance of your current weight as a first step toward making a real and lasting change. The following fantasy may help you to move toward acceptance.

A Fantasy

Imagine that some strange gas has just been injected into the earth's atmosphere. The moment you inhale this gas it becomes impossible for you ever to gain or lose weight again. Not a pound. Not an ounce. Your body will remain in its present shape for the rest of your life.

If you are a chronic dieter it will be terribly difficult for you to allow yourself this fantasy. It means that the game of Change Your Shape and Change Your Life is over. We ask you to let go of your fear long enough to enter the fantasy. Imagine that for the rest of your life your weight will stay exactly as it is right now. Ask yourself what you would do.

Would you continue to berate yourself for your shape once you accept the fantasy that your body will never change? Would you continue to wear uncomfortable clothing if you knew that your weight was not going anywhere? Would you run five miles today? Would you stay away from the beach forever? Would you continue to "feast" on celery and carrot sticks, or would you relax and eat what you want?

Indeed, most compulsive eaters are shocked by their response to this fantasy. They hate to think of a world in which they cannot strive for thinness, but once they imagine themselves there for a little while they begin to feel relaxed. Most people realize that in such an atmosphere they would trade their too-tight clothing for something more comfortable. They'd go to the beach for a swim. They'd stop thinking about what they're supposed to eat and start thinking about what they want to eat. They understand that in this fantasy world they wouldn't feel as anxious as usual. And they notice that if they felt less anxious because they were no longer yelling at themselves about their eating and their shape, they'd eat less.

Our notion of accepting yourself requires that you live as if this fantasy were reality. Remember, we're not suggesting that you resign yourself to being fat but that you acknowledge *what is* without judging that reality. Most compulsive eaters, when confronted with this idea, complain that they would live that way if only they could begin at a much lower weight, as in "Couldn't I diet first and *then* move to this weird planet?" The fact is that living in this fantasy, regardless of the weight at which you enter it, offers one hell of a vacation from the stress of your addiction.

We know, however, that most of you will not be able to live as if you will never lose another pound without first putting up a fight. At the heart of your resistance is the question "How can I accept myself when I really hate myself?"

"How Can I Accept Myself When I Really Hate Myself?"

"It may be," said Ellen, "that you're right. The more I hate myself for eating and the more I tell myself how ugly I am, the more I eat and the worse I feel. Maybe I do have to stop yelling at myself, but how can I? I do think I look terrible at this weight and most of the time I do think my eating is disgusting. I don't even taste what I'm eating. I just stuff my face. How can I like all that? Am I supposed to tell myself that it's fine to devour a whole cake? Am I supposed to lie and tell myself that my fat is beautiful?"

Ellen's questions are right on target. She wants to know how she can possibly accept and live with what she and almost everyone around her regard as unacceptable. No doubt you, too, find it hard to imagine not saying yuck and feeling "yucky" when you look in the mirror, and you certainly can't fathom waking up the morning after a binge without screaming your way into another diet.

We are not suggesting that you must like your body if you don't. We are certainly not suggesting that you must like feeling driven to eat. Liking or not liking something is almost beside the point. Acceptance does not imply self-delusion. It involves coming to terms with what is. When you accept yourself you simply say "This is how I am right now. I don't know what the future will bring. I do know that if I want to change, I must first feel as comfortable as I can with myself in the present."

You eat compulsively and your body reflects both the body type you inherited and the history of your addictive relationship to food. The state of your eating and of your body are neither good nor bad but simply what they are. As you resolve your compulsive eating your body will reflect this change and you will resume what, for you, is a natural weight. For now, however, developing an acceptance of your need to eat and of your body as it exists is crucial to resolving your problem with food.

Moving Toward Acceptance

In order to move toward acceptance you need to remember several things.

Remember that the contempt you feel for your eating and your weight wasn't your idea in the first place. It's something you learned. You are surrounded by constant reminders that thin is better and eating is disgusting. When you hear your-self repeating these messages, remember where you got them. Should you forget, just pick up a magazine or turn on the TV. As long as you remember that these ideas came from "out there," you can return them to their rightful home. You can evaluate these ideas, reject them, and develop your own point of view.

Of course, you would prefer it if everyone else came around to your new way of thinking. Unfortunately, it takes many years for shifts in cultural attitudes to occur, so for the present, you must go it alone, difficult as it is to develop an independent point of view. You must accept and treat your-self the way you've always wished others would. Put more positively, you no longer have to wait for others to accept you as you are. You can start living with yourself in a new way. As you do so, you will feel better and be encouraged to move ahead.

- Remember that your self-hatred is the factor most re-sponsible for keeping you at a miserable standstill. Self-contempt makes you feel bad, and when you feel bad you eat. Each critical remark you make puts you at risk for compulsive eating. The rebel within you will not bow down to your abuse. When you accuse yourself, that rebel takes you directly to the fridge in an attempt to feel better.
- Remember that your driven need to eat and your weight are parts of you that have been resistant to change. Clearly, they have great value and signifi-cance, although they cause you much pain. The logic of your eating may still elude you, but that logic is there nonetheless. Each person, in the course of his or her development, finds ways of integrating and coping with life experiences. Why is your way, eating, either

bad or good? It is simply the way you have found to solve your dilemmas. The more you see your eating as one of many possible ways to cope, the less stigmatized you'll feel.

The Mechanics of Acceptance

Stopping the Thought: "I understand all those things I'm supposed to remember, and I remember them," said Joan, who was struggling with the notion of acceptance. "The problem is that when it comes right down to it, I can't help thinking what I think. I see my reflection in the mirror and I'm horrified."

We know that Joan, and thousands like her, believe that they can't help thinking what they think. For most compulsive eaters, self-flagellation is a reflex reaction. You feel anxious, you eat, and you berate yourself. You call yourself names. You hate yourself. You feel hopeless. You look in the mirror and say "yuck." You don't like what you see and are only beginning to develop an acceptance, albeit a grudging one, of your need to eat.

We know, however, that with experience you can learn to do something about what you think. You *can* notice when you have denigrating thoughts about your eating and your body and once you've noticed such thoughts you can learn to set them aside. Your negative thoughts and feelings about your eating and your body seem to have a life of their own. It is your job to take them in hand.

It's a tricky process, learning to stop your thoughts, one that will take some practice. Step one is to catch yourself in the act of thinking negatively about your eating or your weight, which is hard to do. These thoughts are second nature to you, and as a result it doesn't feel unusual when you have them. Step two involves addressing your negative thoughts directly. You can challenge them with your new awareness about your eating, your weight, and the process of change.

At the moment people have such negative thoughts they think that dwelling on them will lead them to act and finally to change. But have you ever really made a change as a result of such thoughts? You've had them for many years and they've never gotten you anywhere.

Your thoughts about your body are similar to the negative thoughts many people have about various aspects of themselves. Some people focus on the size of their nose; others obsess about their receding hairline; some berate themselves continuously for their procrastination; still others return daily to the theme of what they perceive to be their lack of talent. These ruminations about what's wrong can take up much of a lifetime. They provide a focus for people and a fantasy that if this one thing were corrected life would go well, but they never inspire change. People feel as if they are being productive when they focus on what's wrong. In fact, they are spinning their wheels and thus staying in a rut. Ultimately, what makes it possible to stop your self-contemptuous thoughts is your conviction that they simply do not work.

In our experience, most people are surprised at the number of thoughts they have to put aside once they start observing the way their thoughts flow. Alan reported that he was surprised at how often he caught himself in the act of dumping on himself. "It's true," he reported. "I'm hardly aware of when these thoughts occur, and I must admit that I do have a hard time letting them go. It's almost as if I'm attached to them."

Let's review the process of stopping a thought. You think, "I can't stand the way I look." You notice the thought and remind yourself that it won't get you anywhere productive. "There's no point to this kind of thinking. It just repeats itself endlessly." You then remind yourself of your new way of thinking. "Although I don't like the way I look, I'm trying to come to terms with it. If I keep thinking negatively about myself, I'll feel awful and then I'll need to eat."

The thought will try to come back. When it does, put it aside again. You need to make a pact with yourself that each time a negative thought reasserts itself, you will put it aside and replace it with a nonjudgmental view. For example, Louis caught himself thinking, "God, did I pig out last night." Realizing that he was calling himself a pig, he rephrased it and said, "Boy, did I ever need to overeat last night. Something must have been up."

Stopping your critical thoughts is an ongoing task in the process of becoming more accepting of yourself and your eating. With what do you replace these negative thoughts? We hope with a more understanding and permissive attitude, one that's more conducive to change.

The Words of Acceptance: We have found that people are able to see that self-contempt does not lead to positive change. They're hard pressed, however, to know what to substitute for it. After all, there are no models for an accepting attitude toward compulsive eating and overweight.

What does acceptance sound like? People who accept themselves are both compassionate and realistic. They do not berate themselves about who they are. Instead, they try to look at themselves and strive for a better understanding of what they'd like to change.

Compulsive eaters must have a sympathetic understanding of their problem that they can state to others, as well as to themselves. You might counter the general cultural position that compulsive eating is a sign of self-indulgence and a lack of willpower by saying, "Eating compulsively, in my view, is the way some people try to calm themselves down."

When you're not at all hungry but reach for food anyway, you might say to yourself, "It's a shame that I feel so uncomfortable right now and that food is the only way I know to deal with anxiety and fear."

You'll probably still eat, but you'll be compassionate about your need to do so, and you certainly won't chastise yourself for it afterward. Instead, you may be curious in the aftermath of your eating to figure out what took you to food at that moment.

On the subject of fat or not so fat, an accepting person might say to others, "People come in different shapes and sizes. The body type we prefer varies according to the decade we live in."

Your private thoughts about your body might run, "This is the size of my body right now. I may not like what I see, but this is it for right now, and it may never change. I'm not going to postpone doing the things I want until I lose some weight."

Let's see what these words and thoughts look like in action.

Felice received an invitation to a party, which she was reluctant to accept.

"When I got the invitation," she explained, "I was kind of excited. The invitation was from a college friend whom I hadn't seen in a couple of years, and I knew that lots of the old crowd would be there. My husband had heard all about these people but never met them.

"My excitement didn't last long, however. I've gained close to twenty-five pounds in the last few years and I felt a terrible conflict. I wanted to see my old friends but I couldn't bear being seen by them, given the way I look. I couldn't imagine what I would wear. Nothing fits me anymore. I felt just awful. I stood at my closet, confronted by the indisput-

*able evidence that once I had been thin and now I was fat,
and I hated myself. I realized I had six weeks before the party
and I thought about how much weight I might be able to
lose on a crash diet, but the whole time I was thinking about
it I was stuffing my face with a bag of Oreos. The whole
thing left me feeling helpless.*

*"A few days later an old friend called from out of town to
say that she was coming in for the party and to ask if she
could stay at our house. I lied and said that I thought we'd
be out of town that weekend, but I left the door open by
saying that we wouldn't know for sure until next week. I
haven't even told my husband about the invitation. I feel
sick about it."*

All compulsive eaters can relate to Felice's experience and
her feelings. Many, however, cannot imagine the alternative
that comes with acceptance.

*"When I got the invitation I was kind of excited," says Fe-
lice. "The idea of my husband's meeting all these old friends,
of their meeting him, was especially wonderful. I immediately realized that I look quite different from the last time I
saw all those people and I clutched for a moment. Then I
tried to think it through.*

*"Of course they'll all notice my weight gain. It's very ob-
vious. I'm aware that it's the result of the last few years
having been hard for me in a number of ways. I don't understand it all, but I'm trying to be accepting and tolerant of
my weight. The most that my friends will know is that something has been going on with me. If they think about it,
beyond noticing that I'm fat, they may feel concerned about
me—and so do I!*

*"I thought about what I had hanging in the closet, real-
ized that nothing would fit me and that I'd have to go out*

and get a new outfit. It occurred to me that it was ridiculous to have all of those clothes that I can't wear hanging in my closet. I need new ones. The party is six weeks off. If I get an early enough start shopping I'm sure that I'll find something that I feel good in. I've always been pretty good at putting myself together.

"A few days later an old friend called from out of town to say that she was coming in for the party and to ask if she could stay at our house. It was great hearing from her and I said I'd be delighted to have her as our guest. When I hung up I felt a moment's panic. What will she think when she sees me? To put my mind at ease I picked up the phone immediately and called her back. 'Listen,' I said, 'this may sound odd to you, but I want to tell you that I've gained quite a bit of weight since I saw you last and I look very different. I didn't want to spend the next few weeks worrying about how I'd feel seeing you and letting you know ahead of time helps. I'm trying to approach my weight problem in a new way, by not dumping on myself or trying to hide it anymore. I'd love to talk about it more with you when I see you.' "

In the second version, Felice was as aware of her weight gain as she was in the first. She accepted it, however, and moved on, rather than seizing it as an excuse to dump on herself. Interestingly, when she was accepting, she didn't need a bag of cookies.

Acceptance, in Felice's case, meant recognizing that in recent years she had a need to eat and her weight gain was the evidence of it. Felice also understood that the impulse to turn to food for help was not a criminal act. Essentially, she could say "I wish I could have found a different way to cope with the pressures in my life these last few years, but I couldn't."

Period. End of statement. She acknowledged her need, recognized that it had resulted in her weight gain, and went on with her life.

Once Felice was able to accept herself, she could begin to deal with the way others regarded her. When a well-meaning friend suggested that they go on a diet together, Felice was able to say "Thanks, but I'm not planning to do anything about my weight right now. I've decided to stop doing all the things that haven't worked for me in the past, like dieting. Instead, I'm just going to live with myself at this weight for a while. It sounds strange, I'm sure, but I think I'll have a better chance at resolving my difficulty with food this way and I'm sure I'll lose weight ultimately. I've actually been feeling much more comfortable these days and a lot less driven to eat."

Living in the Present

Shifting from a negative view of your weight and your eating to neutrality and acceptance is a radical transition for any compulsive eater to make, and it involves more than just words. Once you say that you will accept yourself, you need to rearrange your life to reflect that acceptance. This rearrangement generally requires purchasing a mirror, tossing a scale, and cleaning a closet.

Purchasing a Mirror

Facing Up to More Than Your Face: Ask a group of compulsive eaters to speak up if they own a full-length mirror and prepare yourself for silence. If the truth be told, most of them avoid looking at themselves.

"Full-length mirror," one woman said, sounding shocked when we asked. "No way. When I accidentally catch a glance of myself in a shop window, I'm shocked and horrified." "Why would I bring a full-length mirror into my home?" another woman asked. "I try to forget what I look like." "If I lost weight and looked like Cheryl Tiegs," said yet another woman, "I'm sure I'd paper my walls with Mylar. As it is, the mirror on my medicine cabinet shows me all I want to see."

Most people do not look like models. Indeed, most models

look more like some abstract notion of beauty than they do like human beings. More often than not, they have had nose jobs or chin jobs or breast implants, and they usually spend the better part of every day tending to their appearance with exercise or cosmetics.

Unfortunately, vast numbers of people, including most compulsive eaters, spend a great deal of energy *wishing* they looked like someone they're not. Sometimes they're too embarrassed to admit the wish. Sometimes they say it out loud. Regardless, the reluctance to look at yourself in a mirror and see clearly what you look like from head to toe, is the common response to the cultural stereotype, thin is in. For far too many people the experience of looking in the mirror—an experience that ought to be pleasurable or at least uncharged—becomes a torturous exercise in self-loathing. It's time to recapture the pleasure of the mirror that you knew as a child. Children are enchanted by their reflections. The mirror can become a friend as well as a major tool in the development of self-acceptance.

Self-acceptance requires self-knowledge. To accept yourself as you are, you have to know who you are. And to know who you are with respect to body size and shape, you have to own and use a full-length mirror.

Know Thyself: Compulsive eaters have a terrible time knowing what they really look like, particularly from the neck down. "Describe your body," we asked a woman who is five feet eight inches tall, broad shouldered, large breasted, wide around the middle, with rather slim legs. "I'm fat," she replied. "Describe your body," we asked another woman who is five feet tall, has thick calves, thighs, and hips, a narrow waist and small breasts. "I'm fat," she told us.

Compulsive eaters are rarely able to discriminate between the parts of their bodies. Instead, they use the word *fat*, in a tone of anger and dissatisfaction, to describe the whole pack-age. To be sure, their catch-all adjective *fat* is not a simple description but a harsh condemnation.

The truth of the matter is that we're all odd, each with a unique combination of characteristics and peculiarities. Some of us are big, others small. Some people have large thighs, others big buttocks. Some have no waists and some large waists. We are angular, curvaceous, flat, and full. We do not, to be sure, look as though we had stepped off an assembly line. Imagine a world in which all bodies were con-sidered interesting and no one better than another.

You need to be able to see your body in order to appreciate it. You may not like everything you see, but you won't even know what there is to like unless you have a good, long look. That's why mirror work is so important.

We don't want you ever again to be caught off guard when you catch your reflection in a shop window. That is a painful and unnecessary experience. In essence, each time it hap-pens you end up saying "I'm terrible" rather than "Oh, that's me!" "Oh, that's me" requires that you know exactly what you look like and can describe yourself without reproach.

Looking at the Looking Glass: If the only mirror you own is on your medicine cabinet, the time has come to make a pur-chase. You should not have to stand on your bed or a chair every time you want to see a full version of yourself. Your days of straining and stretching are over. The time has come to go out and buy yourself a nondistorting full-length mirror.

Buying a mirror is the first step in seeing what exists. Think about your face for a moment. Our faces are far from uniform and far from the projected ideal of beauty, yet most of us have come to terms with what our faces look like. For some reason, however, most of us have a harder time ac-cepting our bodies than we do our faces.

We accept our faces, in part, because we see them all the time, but we may not look at our bodies in the mirror daily, as we do our faces. Indeed, our faces are very familiar and, more often than not, we are able to talk about them in terms of what we like. "I have nice eyes." "I have a friendly smile." "I like my coloring." What we don't like we learn to live with. We have learned that if you look at your body as routinely and nonjudgmentally as you look at your face, you will be able to feel a similar kind of acceptance.

Once you have purchased your full-length mirror you'll have to figure out where to put it, which may take some thought. The purpose of owning a mirror is to see yourself, to develop a real sense of your body. The mirror work we suggest is best done in privacy when other demands are not being made of you. You should hang your mirror in a place that best offers the quiet opportunity to look.

Once you are ready to look you'll need to remind yourself of the meaning of acceptance. The goal of all mirror work is to be able to see yourself *without uttering one negative word*. If you're not accustomed to looking in the mirror, this assignment will be difficult. We suggest that you start slowly.

Take a few minutes each day to look at yourself. Imagine that you are an artist describing a piece of sculpture. You want to be able to describe yourself without making any judgments. Start at the top of your head and make your way down to your toes. "I am round here, but long there. I'm very smooth here and rough and hairy there. I go out here but get flatter down there." The moment you hear yourself say something negative or begin to judge what you see is the moment to step away from your reflection. When the judgment begins, the mirror work ends. Tomorrow you'll begin again.

If you do this exercise for a few minutes every day, you will eventually learn what your body looks like. As you begin to feel more comfortable with what you see, you may even want to touch yourself to feel your parameters. At some point you will become as comfortable looking at yourself without your clothing on as you are when your body is covered. The goal is to be able to expand the vocabulary with which you describe yourself to move from judgments like "fat" to genuine description. It's a most attainable goal.

Tossing a Scale

"The first thing I do every morning is get on my scale," explained Maryann, a woman in her mid-thirties who has spent the last twelve years attempting to control her weight and eating. "I'm always a little nervous just before I step on, and it's no wonder. For me, the scale has a lot of power. If I see that I've lost a few pounds I feel great. I think about eating breakfast or calling up a client and making a lunch date. I go to my closet and pick out something bright or slinky to wear to work. I leave my house in a good mood, confident that my day will go well.

"If, when I step on that scale, I find that I've gained any weight," Maryann continued, "even if it's less than a pound, I get depressed. Sometimes I hop on and off, trying to rearrange my feet so the weight will change. I even push the scale to a different corner of my bathroom and get on again. I've got all these little tricks to shave off an ounce or two. But if it happens that I weigh more than I did the day before, I feel awful. I think about everything I ate in the last twenty-four hours. I skip breakfast and vow to miss lunch as well. I approach my closet with dread and pick out things that are dark and baggy. And I head out of my house feeling fat and in a lousy mood."

Maryann is not alone. Every day, millions of people allow their bathroom scales to determine their general outlook. Most of us who live in a fat-phobic culture are addicted to the scale. When our weight is high, we feel low; when it's low, we feel high. We allow the scale to tell us how we're doing with regard to much more than weight.

If you are earnest about accepting yourself, the scale must go. Simply put, the scale is the most powerful symbol of nonacceptance in your life. It measures and it judges. It sits quietly in a corner of your bathroom and beckons. "Come on. What harm can I do? Take a chance. Maybe you'll get good news."

Acceptance means recognizing that good news from the scale is just as damaging as bad news. If the scale gives you good news it is actually telling you that you were unacceptable yesterday. If the scale gives you bad news, it's saying that you are unacceptable today. Acceptance means that you acknowledge what your body looks like without berating yourself. When you get rid of your scale once and for all, you are basically saying "I won't allow the numbers on that scale to continue to torment me." You are stating that you will no longer tolerate an external judge's telling you how good or bad you've been.

"But how will I know what's happening with my weight?" Maryann asked. The answer is that your eyes will tell you what is happening to your body. You can also see what's happening by the fit of your clothes. More to the point, compulsive eaters generally know their weight within an ounce at any given moment.

Once you get rid of your scale your vision will become considerably more acute. "When I weighed myself every morning and night," said Arlene, "I really believed the scale above myself. If I woke up feeling pretty good about myself and the scale told me I had gained a pound, I'd start to feel bad. If I put on something that I had saved for my thin days, but then discovered that I weighed more than I thought, I'd take it off. No matter how good I thought it looked on me before, once I got the scale's verdict, it began to look bad."

Without the scale, you can see how things really fit. You can decide for yourself whether or not something looks good on you. You can feel for yourself if your clothing is too loose or too tight. You'll know about changes in your body because you'll see and feel them.

Occasionally, a compulsive eater has a negative reaction to throwing away the scale. It has become a part of such people, and asking them to throw it away is like asking them to cut off an arm. "When I set my two feet on the scale and watch the numbers," Alice told us, "I feel very substantial. The scale tells me that I exist." If you experience the scale this way, go easy. See what happens as you begin to dress differently and eat differently. These changes alone will lead to new feelings of self-acceptance and a firmer sense of your existence.

For those of you who can't bear the idea of throwing your scale away for good, we urge you to put it out of reach, where you won't see it. Pack it up and store it in the back of a closet. The scale is a weight watcher's most valuable tool. Once you become not-a-weight-watcher, and once your ability to see yourself sharpens, the scale's importance will diminish.

Cleaning a Closet

How many selves are hanging in your closet? The closets of compulsive eaters reflect their aspirations, their anguish, and their compromises. More important, the closets of compulsive eaters say much about their history and almost nothing about their present. While others throw away what they haven't used in a year or two, compulsive eaters never dare throw anything away. Their past is always their future. They always think "Maybe I'll get into this again some day" or "If I gain back my weight I'll need this." Adele, at twenty-five, cannot remember a time when she felt genuinely good about her body.

"Basically, I have three wardrobes hanging in my closet. There's my skinny clothing, most of which I bought several years ago after two months on the Scarsdale diet. I see that stuff every morning and feel like crying. It's so tiny, I can't believe I ever got into it. How could I have allowed myself to go from that thin to this fat? And then there's my fat clothing. That's the stuff I have to wear when I'm at my worst. It's good for me to look at it, even though it makes me feel sick, because it's a warning for me. If I don't watch it I'll be wearing those muumuus again. And then, of course, there's my in-between clothing, the stuff that fits me when I'm not at my fattest or my thinnest. I'd say about half the things in that category are pretty nice, and the rest are things I make do with."

What we suggest is that Adele, and everyone else with three wardrobes, begin a major cleaning effort, the goal of which is to rid your closet of everything that doesn't fit. All that should remain are the things that both fit you and appeal to you. Take the clothes that are too small and either throw them out or pack them up and put them in the basement. Remember, accepting yourself the way you are means not yelling at yourself about your body. Going to the closet each morning and finding clothing that doesn't fit is a painful experience and a form of daily self-criticism. Adele was clearly saying that her skinny self was her better self.

It may be hard for you to let go of the skinny clothing because it represents hope and the fat clothing because it represents safety. But chances are that the clothing you are saving for your future body will be out of style by the time you get to wear it. If it hurts too much to give it away, pack it away for safekeeping.

Once you've disposed of everything that doesn't fit, go through what is left. This time, weed through the clothes and decide whether you like them. Ask yourself if your wardrobe is representative of your taste. When you wake in the morning, will you feel good about what you see in your closet? Feeling good about what's hanging there at any given moment is an expression of your acceptance. The chances are that most of you will have very little left once you've cleaned out your closet. You've been living with closets filled with "not me." Now that your closet is empty, the time has come to shop.

Before you go shopping, however, think about what kind of clothing you'd like to wear. A shopping trip can be very uncomfortable for someone who has a history of hating his or her body, so we suggest that you ease into it. Look through some fashion magazines. Allow yourself to fantasize about the kind of clothing you like. What kinds of fabric do you find most appealing? What colors are most flattering to you? Most important, how do you want to look right now, as opposed to twenty pounds from now?

When you're ready to look at what's available, make certain to go to a store with a large selection and give yourself time. No one is standing over your shoulder with a gun, telling you to buy. Get the lay of the land. Experiment in the dressing room. Try on as much as you want, or don't try on anything. Your first trip out might just be a look-and-see. It isn't time to buy until you're entirely comfortable and you see precisely what you want.

A word of caution. Do not look at sizes. Look at the garments, find them in whatever size fits, and buy them if you like the way they look. Size tickets are like scales. Many compulsive eaters have actually cut the size labels out of their clothing because they make them feel so embarrassed. Just use your eyes and your body to figure out what you'd like to wear, and remember that the goal is comfort and looking good, no matter what your size. You no longer need to wear clothing that's tight as a reminder that you should lose weight or in the hope that someday soon it will fit. Dressing for now means that comfort and style go together.

People hearing this often tell us how difficult it is to have nice clothing when you're a large size. It is true that most designers cater to people who are very thin. That situation is changing somewhat, but once you accept that large is large, not bad, you will be able to find creative ways to put together a terrific wardrobe.

Nancy Roberts, radio host, author, actress, and model, started dieting at the age of eight. She's been up and down in weight throughout her life. She is a very large woman who decided some years ago that the time had come to say no more diets, no more self-contempt, and no more waiting to live life in a thinner body. She dresses beautifully with a great deal of style and personal flair. She is a model for all of us who live a life of "if only," a life spent waiting to live. Nancy has made her story available to all of us in her aptly titled book, *Breaking All the Rules*.

* * *

Once you've hung your mirror, tossed your scale, and cleaned your closet, you're ready to go about your life. If you've wanted to take a dance class but were too afraid to do it until you were thinner, now is the time to enroll. What about the vacation you've always wanted to take in the sun but didn't because you were reluctant to wear light and revealing clothing?

In the past you've used your weight as a reason for not

doing many things. Once you accept yourself as you are, you have a choice about what you want to do. If you've said, "If only I were thinner, I'd apply for a better position," you need to evaluate your situation independently of your shape. Do you or don't you want to make a move? If you want to but are afraid, what's really standing in your way? If you've said, "If only I were thin, I would go to the beach," you need to think about how you could make yourself comfortable on the beach as you are. When you accept yourself, you no longer allow your weight to determine what you do or don't do. You declare yourself as entitled to life as anyone else.

– 7 –

Dumping the Diet

Living in the present—substituting self-acceptance for negative judgments—is the first step you must take toward freeing yourself from compulsive eating. Your condemnation of your eating and the size of your body has always led you to diet. The diet has been the restraint you've imposed on yourself as a punishment for "not looking right." It has been an instrument of self-hatred. Therefore, the next major step you must take toward freeing yourself is to say *no more diets!*

Impossible as it may seem to you to abandon diets, if you review your experience with them and consider the data we've presented, you'll bolster your faltering resolve. Remember:

1. Ninety-eight percent of dieters regain their weight plus some.
2. Diets make you fat.
3. Deprivation ensures a fight-back response—the binge.

The resolution never to diet again cannot hinge on whether you feel thin or fat, on whether you have a big party or a job interview coming up, or on the advent of summer, fall, winter, or spring. Until you promise yourself that you are finished with diets—grapefuit diets, papaya diets, protein

diets, carbohydrate diets, eat-all-you-want diets, and starvation diets—you will not be in a position to end your food
obsession. The way you feel about food will not change until
you say "That's it. I've spent the better part of my life dieting
and, whether I lose or gain weight, I will never again deprive
myself of food. I'm finished with diets forever."

This declaration, despite its logic, is perhaps the most difficult statement a compulsive eater will ever make. All compulsive eaters—even the enlightened ones—fear that without the restrictions of a diet they will devour the world. "I'll
start eating and never stop." "I'll get to be as big as a house."
"I may end up in the same place every year, but if I didn't
put the brakes on every now and then I'd really blow up."

Let us reassure you that every compulsive eater feels this
fear when faced with the prospect of giving up diets. Those
people who've had it with dieting and can take this step feel
more relaxed, more in control, and eat considerably less than
they ever thought possible. After a lifetime of attempting to
control yourself, however, it's reasonable to expect an intense reaction and a mixed bag of emotions once you consider stepping away from the diet. Ready yourself for feelings
that run the gamut from giddiness to terror to sadness and
finally to relief.

Giddiness

Whenever we introduce the idea of never dieting again,
people laugh nervously, as if someone had suggested doing
something naughty. Much of your life has been spent monitoring everything you put in your mouth. You're always
either on or off a diet, and each mouthful is judged accordingly. We are suggesting that, for the first time, you not be
on or off a diet but that you simply be. There's a headiness
that comes with the taste of such freedom. You feel off balance at first, but intrigued.

"Are you really telling me that I should just eat anything I want?" Helene asked us. "You obviously don't know me very well." Then she began to laugh, and her laughter was met with more laughter from the group. None of them could imagine a life without food rules. The prospect was titillating, as dangerous things can be. For most people, however, the sense of danger quickly overrides the excitement.

Terror

You will never diet again, and you are terrified. Your terror makes sense. Until now your only frame of reference for eating without restraints has been binging. You binged and felt completely out of control; now that you've sworn off your most familiar symbol of control, the diet, you have those same out-of-control feelings. You feel as though eating without restraints and binging are the same thing. No more diets translates, in the mind of a lifelong dieter, into a lifelong binge. Given that binging is always accompanied by inner chaos, followed by fat and feelings of self-loathing, it's no wonder that the notion of a lifelong binge sets your teeth on edge.

What you forget is that in the past you'd never made a conscious, purposeful decision *not to diet.* When you went out of control you were actually on the last lap of the diet/binge cycle, simply *reacting* to your self-imposed constraints by breaking out. When you ate a dozen doughnuts, your motivation had more to do with stuffing it all in while off the diet than with a genuine desire for doughnuts. Binging is a negative reaction to the deprivation of diets that has nothing to do with what you really want.

Abandoning diets, on the other hand, is an affirmative action rooted in your desire to get in touch with your real needs and appetites, and it puts you in new territory. Although you may feel out of control when you first abandon diets—a frightening feeling with which we feel great sympathy—you have to ride out your fear before you can begin to hope for self-regulation. When you have eliminated all the shoulds and should nots that have been attached to your eating, you will feel much more in control around food.

Skeptical? We have found that people who take a chance on giving up diets eat excessively for only as long as they hedge their bets. Giving up diets, however, is a bold step to take. Understandably, people do hedge their bets and when they do, they get into trouble.

Fred thought that what we said about the diet/binge cycle made sense and decided to try to give up diets. After a week of "no diets" he began to panic. "Every night I come home with ice cream and cookies and Chinese food and I eat and eat and eat. I've gained five pounds this week and I can't imagine going on at this rate. The problem is that when I have food in the house I feel compelled to eat it. I can't put away a half-eaten pint of ice cream."

We soon discovered that although Fred had said he would give up diets, he was really approaching the whole project as an experiment. What he was doing was trying out giving up diets. He'd bring home the foods he wanted to eat and watch himself to see what happened. He'd sit down with a book and think about his ice cream. He'd take it out of the freezer, eat a dishful, return to his book, and think again about his ice cream. He'd get another dishful and continue this way until he'd finished it off.

Fred was out to see how well he could resist the food he brought home. Resisting, however, has more to do with diets than with dumping diets. Essentially, Fred was saying that he would stop dieting only if he proved to himself that he could have food in the house and not eat it—"I'll stop dieting if you can assure me I won't eat compulsively."

Such assurances are impossible. Fred has been a compulsive eater for most of his life. Dumping diets is only a first step on the way to resolving compulsive eating. Until he genuinely does away with his restrictions, Fred will continue to feel compelled to react against them.

After some denial, Fred admitted that, rather than making a commitment to dumping diets, he had only been trying the notion on for size. He had not really decided never again to deprive himself of food. He had taken on the task of dumping diets as though it was a new diet. He figured that he'd have food around for a while and see what happened, knowing full well that if it didn't work, he'd go back on a diet.

Unfortunately, Fred's attempts to resist food only exacerbated his compulsive eating. As long as the rebel within Fred knew that having a well-stocked freezer was a temporary indulgence, it was going to get what it could while the getting was good.

Sandra had a more successful experience than Fred. She took the chance and saw that when you dump the diet you no longer crave foods the same way. "I don't think my diets have been very serious for a long time now. Sure, I've gone on diets and off them, but somewhere I think I've recognized that diets have never really done me much good. So I really was ready for someone to come along and tell me to dump them."

During her first few weeks of active nondieting Sandra kept her cupboard stocked with cookies. "I would never have thought this possible," she said at the end of three weeks, "but I've several half-eaten boxes of cookies on my shelves. I can't believe it. For the first time in my life I don't feel as though I have to eat the whole box. It's the strangest thing, but I'm not really trying to keep myself away from them. Of course, I went through a lot of boxes of cookies before I got used to having them in the house, but I kept buying more and at some point began to notice that I was eating them less.

"Basically, I'm eating whatever I want, whenever I want it, without giving it much thought. It feels great not to be watching myself all the time. I don't think I'm eating *that* much, but I do worry about what's going to happen to my weight if I make cookies a way of life."

The terror of dumping diets is, ultimately, the terror of losing control and gaining weight. Regardless of what we say, and regardless of what you have come to know, it's hard to give up the belief that diets keep your weight down.

We have made the point that dieting, in and of itself, is often responsible for making us fat. When you diet your metabolism slows down and preserves fat. Consequently, each successive diet must be more extreme in order for you to lose the same amount of weight. Some people maintain artificially thin bodies—bodies they were not genetically programmed to have—by living in a constant and ever increasing state of deprivation. Few people, however, can maintain an artificially thin body indefinitely. Most people maintain a mean weight as a result of the endless diet/binge cycle. As a result, once they stop hedging and make a firm commitment to dumping the diet, they are surprised to discover that their weight simply stays where it is. It may go up a bit until they are convinced that the food is here to stay, but it will go down once they resolve the compulsive quality of their eating.

You and your body are self-regulatory. You are going to learn how to let your body tell you how it should be fed, and in the process many of you will also lose weight. We recognize, however, that you haven't yet accepted the idea that you can self-regulate and that stopping dieting is a frightening step for you to take. From your perspective, the possiblity of gaining even a few pounds seems intolerable.

We see again and again that those people who stop dieting and are able to stop scolding themselves for eating see immediately that they actually eat less. It is essential to remember that *scolding and weight gain go hand in hand*. If you let go of the rules and do not yell at yourself about food, you will eat less compulsively. Giving up diets is liberating. It can also be quite sad.

Sadness

Dieting, as we've said, provides the hope that by altering our bodies we can alter the way we feel about ourselves and our lives. We think about dieting to make ourselves feel better when we feel bad and to provide a solution to myriad problems. When we stop dieting we relinquish hope of a magical change and feel sad.

Mary heard us out with an open mind. After a while she could see that dieting and its attendant self-contempt had made her fat; barring one problem, she was ready to stop. "My problem is that summer's coming," Mary said. "Everything you've presented makes sense to me, but when I think about going through another summer in my body I feel very sad. I can't face the idea of going out on a beach at this weight. Just once I'd like to feel okay for summer. How about if I lose some weight first and then give up dieting?"

People laughed because they all wanted to do exactly the same thing: lose weight first, then deal with their eating problem. No matter how often experience shows us that we spring back to our familiar shape at the end of each diet, we cling to the fantasy that with enough willpower we can make a permanent change. Mary knew that dumping diets meant giving up the hope that she could be different, more beautiful, and less self-conscious in time for summer. It meant accepting that for the foreseeable future she'd have to remain at her present size. The realization left her feeling unexpectedly and overwhelmingly sad.

It is sad to give up the fantasy of "fitting in in thirty days." We have all used this fantasy to lift our spirits when we feel low. Like Mary, we've imagined ourselves walking on the beach in a different body, and for a moment we've felt better. It's hard to let go of that. But fantasies are just that—they're not life. The game of Change Your Shape and Change Your Life keeps you from living your life in the present.

It's also hard for people to let go of the fantasy that dieting will solve all their problems, and we call this fantasy into play more often than we know. Compulsive eaters reach for food whenever they feel uncomfortable, and each time they do they have the fantasy that if they could keep themselves from doing it, that is, stay on a diet, life wouldn't be as tough.

After a week of "not dieting," Richard reported that he had mixed feelings about it. "It was a tremendous relief not to be *on* a diet," he said, "and you were right. My eating did slow down. I was very surprised about that. I even left some food on my plate at a restaurant the other night. I haven't done that in twenty years. But I noticed that I felt kind of depressed. For the first time in as long as I can remember, I wasn't obsessed with food or with dieting. What happened, however, was that I became more aware than ever of all the problems I face every day. I guess I really was spending a lot of energy distracting myself from those problems by focusing on what I was eating. It's depressing to think about how many problems I have to solve. I hope that if I can get the eating out of the way, I'll be in better shape to deal with life in general."

People feel sad about the loss of diets as a magical solution to many problems. Compulsive eaters also feel sad and concerned about giving up dieting because it represents a way of life. It's strange but true that people whose lives have been organized around a particular difficulty feel a similar sense of loss when the problem is resolved. For example, people with chronic pain sometimes find themselves depressed once it's gone.

Compulsive eaters like Richard have spent their lives preoccupied with their need for food and what to do about it. This obsession has enveloped them. The diet has been their constant companion, seducing them with the "if only" of thinness. Losing that companionship—as unpleasant and uncomfortable as it may be—is a loss. A couple unhappily married for twenty years usually feels some loss along with relief when they finally split up. So it is with compulsive eaters and diets.

Christina put it best when she said, "I'm worried that if I stop thinking about dieting I'll have all this time on my hands. It's true that I hate being constantly preoccupied with what I eat, but it's a very big part of my life. I feel as if I'm about to jump into a void."

Relief

Terror and sadness are ubiquitous reactions to our suggestion to stop dieting. But it's not long before people report feeling relief. What's often unclear to people who have developed a ritual like compulsive eating—which is an attempt to deal with pain—is that the pain they are trying to avoid is ultimately less painful than the ritual itself. We start avoiding pain early in life, and many of us never stop to reevaluate our circumstances. What is painful and overwhelming in childhood is rarely so in adulthood. Therefore, most people when they stop dieting and scolding themselves for eating are surprised to find that life is much easier than they anticipated.

Karen, at forty-five, had been riding the diet/binge cycle since she was a teenager, and the ongoing effort had worn her down. She found some comfort in the notion that her problems with diets had more to do with diets than with her own inadequacy, and the suggestion that her eating habits were an act of rebellion against the culture gave her some relief, some respite from her self-contempt. Indeed, those two notions—the foundation of our suggestion that she finally dump the diet—offered Karen enough hope to enable her to take a chance.

Karen went to the supermarket and bought everything that appealed to her. "I walked up and down the aisles and pretended I was *normal*," Karen told us. "I just bought whatever I wanted and didn't think about whether it was fattening or what the checkout clerk would think about the contents of my cart.

"When I got home I opened several pints of ice cream and ate quite a bit, but I bought so much that even *I* couldn't think about finishing it all. When I went to sleep that night there was still lots of ice cream left. It was a strange feeling because I'd usually buy one pint and stuff it all in. This time I bought six pints and had less of an urge to gorge myself."

When Karen woke up the next morning, she remembered what she had eaten the night before. She felt anxious and guilty, but she didn't rush desperately to the refrigerator in an attempt to deal with her feelings. Instead, she remembered that she'd promised herself never to go on another diet, no matter what happened. Therefore, she tried not to condemn herself for last night's ice cream as she would have done in the past, nor did she put herself on a get-rid-of-last-night's-ice-cream diet.

Karen ate a lot during that week, but far less than she would have expected. "I can't believe it," she said. "I get up every morning, think about grabbing something to eat, go to the cupboard, and relax. I have lots of food around and, much to my surprise, that makes me feel secure. It's still hard for me to think that I may never be as thin as I've always longed to be, and it's clear that I'm not going to lose all my weight in a month. I feel upset about that, but I can't get over how relieved I feel each time I remember that I'm not dieting."

Karen took a big chance and, as a result, made some important discoveries. She promised herself that she would never again deprive herself of food. She stopped calling herself fat and bad. When she stopped focusing on what her life would be like *if* she were thin, Karen saw a real change in the driven quality of her eating.

Karen was fed up with the diet/binge cycle and willing to do whatever was necessary to end her obsession with eating and weight. She was able to remind herself, each time she reached for formerly forbidden foods, that whatever happened, she would never again diet. Each time she reminded herself that she had dumped the diet, she was able to relax. And the more she relaxed, the less drawn to food she felt.

Karen and all compulsive eaters who stop dieting are headed on a new path. They say no more diets and no more contempt in order to establish the basis for a new kind of eating, namely, demand feeding. Although giving up dieting is a frightening step to take, people are able to stick with it because they immediately discover how much better they feel free of diets. They are amazed to find that they feel more in control, more relaxed, and more hopeful than ever about finally resolving this painful problem.

– 8 –

Living Free in a World of Food

The most important prerequisite for curing compulsive eating is to stop dieting. However, no one who has been involved in a long-term battle with compulsive eating can be expected to declare a lasting moratorium on diets without help in developing a totally new attitude toward food.

Compulsive eaters assume that food is their problem. Our contention is that food is *not* the problem. Compulsive eaters use food for anxiety rather than for the purpose it is designed to serve, the satisfaction of physiological hunger. Misuse of food cannot be corrected until compulsive eaters make peace with food itself. We call this process "legalizing." Living free in a world of food is the foundation for demand feeding.

Carrot Sticks versus Carrot Cake

Compulsive eaters are engaged in an ongoing struggle with food, and it's no wonder. Food frightens them. Food thrills them. Food offers them satisfaction. And food renders them helpless. Indeed, their love/hate relationship with food consumes them.

If you are a compulsive eater, you have probably spent much of your life attempting to avoid food. The first step in combating your obsession with food and weight, then, is to put an end to this avoidance. Dumping the diet means, fundamentally, that you will never again think of any food as "fattening" or "forbidden."

The notion of forbidden food runs very deep. Chronic and periodic dieters alike never question the idea that some foods are allowed, harmless, and not fattening, while others are forbidden, fattening, and sinful. The calorie chart long ago became fixed in the mind of each compulsive eater.

"I try to keep lots of carrot sticks in my fridge," Midge told us, "so that when I feel that I need to nosh on something I've got them handy." "Are carrot sticks what you really feel like eating when you have the urge to nosh?" we asked. Midge looked at us incredulously, then laughed. "Of course not. What sane person ever gets an overwhelming urge for a carrot stick. But they're healthy and have hardly any calories, and at this point I don't really mind them."

We asked Midge to think about what foods she'd like to have in her refrigerator if she didn't have to think about words like *calories, healthy,* and *fattening.* "That's a hard one," she answered quite honestly. Midge has been forbidding herself foods for so long that it takes some real effort to think about just what foods she might want to have around. Finally she said, "Right now, maybe because I was talking about carrots, what comes to mind is carrot cake, with that cream cheese and sugar frosting, lots of thick frosting."

The time had come for Midge to stop making the usual distinction between carrot sticks and carrot cake and start making peace with the foods she had not allowed herself to have. We suggested that on her way home she buy three carrot cakes with cream cheese and sugar frosting—one as a backup for the freezer—instead of just one, because we could anticipate that Midge, who had spent years depriving herself of such cake, might need to eat a great deal of it to convince herself that carrot cake would, in the future, always be there for her.

This impulse to eat lots of foods that have been forbidden in the past is a compulsive eater's way of saying "Pinch me. Am I dreaming?" But once you are convinced that these foods are there to stay, you won't feel the need to eat as much of them. This, of course, is the underlying key to our program, and it is almost impossible for any compulsive eater to believe. Your acceptance and conviction will grow only as you take the chance and legalize food yourself.

Legalizing Food

Legalizing food means, quite simply, that you allow yourself to have the foods you want—nothing is forbidden. Binging and dieting are simply two sides of the same coin. Legalizing foods—removing all the taboos, restrictions, and external controls with regard to your eating—is the way out of the diet/binge cycle.

Once you have legalized food, you will never again forbid yourself any foods. You won't eat carrot sticks because they are low in calories when you really want carrot cake. You won't eat carob when you crave chocolate. You won't eat frozen yogurt when you want double-rich Häagen-Dazs ice cream. You will be free to eat what you want, when you want it. And in time you will discover that what you really want may not be what you think you would want if you were free to eat as you please.

The way to demonstrate to yourself that there are no foods on your restricted list is to make sure that all the foods you like are available and abundant. This issue of plentitude is very important. When you bring the foods you love into your home, you need to have them around in sufficient quantity so that the amount you eat will never be determined by the amount in your cupboard. You are going to prove to yourself that you really mean business. You will surround yourself with your favorite foods, eat them when you want them, and most important, not berate yourself when you've finished, no matter how much you've eaten.

Until now you have clung to aphorisms like "out of sight, out of mind," even though you know, in your heart of hearts, that every time you remove yourself from the foods you desire, your desire for them is heightened. Tell yourself that you cannot have cheesecake for six months, and chances are that every day of those six months you will think about cheesecake. You'll look at a menu and your eyes will become riveted on *cheesecake*. You'll open a magazine and be faced with an advertisement for cheesecake. Everything around you will trigger thoughts of cheesecake.

Food bans create an exaggerated yearning. When is the last time you found yourself dreaming about a salad with no dressing? There's no getting around the fact that a piece of naked lettuce doesn't have the allure of a hot fudge sundae. Once you legalize foods, however, and lift all the bans, once you declare that nothing is fattening, bad, forbidden, or off limits, you defuse all of the artificially induced cravings and begin to get in touch with what foods you really desire. Sometimes you'll want cake and sometimes you'll want carrot sticks. Once cake is legal, you'll have the freedom to choose.

Eventually, all your food choices will be based on what and how much your body needs. Our natural physiological mechanisms are self-regulatory. As you'll see later, studies have shown that young babies, left to their own devices, will choose all the foods they need to ensure healthy growth and development. Before you put food into your mouth you must simply ask yourself "Am I hungry?" If the answer is yes, the question that naturally follows is "What are you hungry for?" You don't think about calories. You don't think about carbohydrates. You don't think about fat. You just think about what you feel like eating and go for it.

Implicit in the act of legalizing foods is the concept of "equalizing foods." This means that ice cream is no better or worse than spinach. Cauliflower has no greater value than pasta or cookies; desserts are the same as main dishes; and so on. We understand, of course, that foods do have different nutritional values and affect each person differently once absorbed in the body, but what we are suggesting is that you make food equal in a psychological sense.

It may sound to you as if we're recommending that you simply go wild and eat everything in sight, but this is not the case. The whole notion of legalizing food is based on the knowledge that once you allow yourself to have, you will want considerably less. It's quite different to say "I want chocolate cake" when chocolate cake is not a special food than to want it because it's forbidden. Difficult as it may be for you to believe, there will come a time when you will be offered a piece of chocolate cake and hear yourself say "No thanks. I'm not really in the mood for that right now."

To Market, To Market . . .

The time has come to make what may be your most memorable trip to the supermarket. Having made the decision to legalize foods, you must take the next step, which is to bring these foods into your home.

The List: Before you go to the market, you have to make a shopping list. Because you have legalized foods, this list will look very different from others you've made in your life. It will be filled with all the things you love to eat but have always feared. There is no need to stock up on sprouts and celery, though we believe the time will come when those foods find their way back on to your lists, not because you *should* eat them but because you *want to*. Most of you are at peace with sprouts and celery. Now you need to fill your cupboards with the foods that you've always longed for but rarely dared to take home. You have to make your peace with food and learn to live with your desires.

What do you love to eat? Do you crave crusty breads and soft sweet rolls? Or are you a chocoholic? Chocolate chocolate chip ice cream with bittersweet hot fudge? What is your fantasy of the perfect meal? Thick lamb chops, mashed potatoes and gravy, blueberry pie à la mode? Or does your taste run more to lasagna, Italian bread with butter, cannoli, and cappuccino? What about those milk shakes you used to drink as a kid? You can buy the same syrup your corner candy store used and make them at home, using more syrup or less, depending on your taste. You can experiment. Indeed, you *should* experiment.

This shopping list, more than any you've ever made, should provide you with the raw material for lots of experimentation. Make sure, however, that you take your time and be as specific as you possibly can. If, for example, you want to buy a bag of candy bars that you loved when you were ten, make certain to get the specific candy bar that you're thinking of. If you have a craving for Snickers, Baby Ruth won't do the trick.

It's not unusual for people to feel anxious while they write their list. Remember, you're committing to paper the names of your most formidable enemies with the intention of bringing them into your home. Allow yourself to feel anxious, but don't allow your anxiety to dictate your list. This is not a prescription for eating everything in sight; it is a serious proposal for confronting fears and taboos and getting beyond them.

Enough Is Not Enough: The issue of quantity is integral to the process of legalizing. Scarcity makes people anxious; surplus creates a sense of well-being and relaxation, the state of mind necessary to feed yourself in an attuned way.

The key to the issue of quantity is to figure out how much of any given food you could possibly eat, then buy more. In the past you defined your appetite by what was on your shelf. If you had a pint of ice cream, you ate a pint of ice cream. Your solution to the problem of wanting to eat everything was to keep your cupboards bare. When we ask compulsive eaters to tell us what's in their refrigerators, they often answer sadly, "Nothing." The time has come to surround yourself with more than you could ever possibly eat.

Imagine, for a moment, that you live in an ice cream parlor. All the ice cream, every bin in every flavor, is there for you. What happens? At first you would probably be very anxious. The thought occurs to you that you might eat and eat and never come up for air. On day one you do eat an extraordinary amount of ice cream. By the end of the day you've eaten about two quarts. Day two might be very much the same.

On day three, however, you have a different feeling—you simply don't want as much ice cream. You're tired of it. The ice cream is there, and you know you can have it whenever you want it, but the question becomes "Do I want it?" That, of course, is a much different question from "May I have it?" The philosophy of architect Mies van der Rohe was "less is more." The philosophy for compulsive eaters should be "more is less—eventually." You have to convince yourself that food is not to be feared, and you do that by creating an environment in which you cannot feel deprived.

Every dieter knows the Sunday-night-eat-it-all-up syndrome. When you are anticipating a famine—diet—on Monday, it makes perfect sense to stoke up on Sunday. In the past, you used the Sunday night feast as evidence of your inability to live amid food. You are ready, now, however, to see what life is like in the ice cream parlor or bakery or candy store—or all three. You will discover that once you are certain you'll never again be faced by a famine, you'll have no need to stoke up.

Ellen has always had a problem with potato chips, her problem being that she loves them. When confronted with a bowl of potato chips, she eats a bowl of potato chips. When confronted with two bags of potato chips, she eats two bags of potato chips. It came as no surprise to find potato chips at the top of Ellen's legalizing list. She had a hard time, however, figuring out how many bags to buy. Finally, she wrote down the number eight and promised herself that when she noticed her supply dwindle to four bags, she'd buy another four.

Henry loves bread. When he thought about his list, he thought about bread. His dreams about bread, however, had nothing to do with the bread one finds on a supermarket shelf. He wanted bakery bread, still warm from the oven. So he decided to make a special trip to his local bakery to buy the bread—one loaf of fresh brown bread with raisins, one loaf of onion rye. While he was thinking about bakery bread it occurred to him that he wanted butter—not salty butter but a tub of the sweet butter his grandmother used to have. He added two pounds of butter to his list and began to feel giddy. He hadn't bought anything but diet margarine since childhood.

Again, it's important to understand that the reason for buying in quantity is not gluttony but to demonstrate to yourself a point that is crucial to your future well-being— that you are never going to deprive yourself of any food again. If you bring home ten boxes of cookies and go through four of them in one night, you go back to the supermarket the next day and replenish your supply. The hard but essential part of this exercise is that you must refill your cupboard without saying one harsh word to yourself about the amount you consumed the night before. When you eat formerly forbidden foods—as you must to reassure yourself that they are legal—you will be tempted to scold yourself and banish the foods from the house forever. It will help you to remember the simple truth that deprivation and scarcity always increase desire. If you keep supplying yourself with surplus, we know that in time you will no longer feel driven to eat.

If in some corner of your mind you have reservations and are secretly telling yourself that you are going to try stocking the house for a week and see what happens, you will inevitably binge and gain weight. You will have turned the process of legalizing food into nothing more than a new diet plan.

When Rita decided to legalize foods, she focused on Ritz crackers and peanut butter, smooth Peter Pan peanut butter. She put "3 jars peanut butter" and "5 boxes Ritz crackers" on her list. When she got home, she sat down and ate a box of crackers and much of a jar of peanut butter. By the next morning she'd eaten another box of crackers and made her way into the second jar of peanut butter. Instead of going out to replace what she'd eaten, Rita began to panic about her weight. She squelched the panic and went back to the market for five more boxes of crackers and three jars of peanut butter.

On the way home Rita couldn't stop thinking about her weight. Starting to think of legalizing food as an experiment, she wasn't too optimistic about the results. She came home and began to polish off her new supply, lecturing herself the way she always had in the past. Her spirits plummeted each time she tossed an empty Ritz box into the trash. All her old feelings came forward. How could she lose weight by "pigging out"?

At that point Rita stopped thinking about replenishing her supplies and thought instead of getting through what she had. The familiar negative voices were getting louder and louder. "When I've finished with all this I'll go on a diet," she thought remorsefully. So she ate, hating herself more with every bite.

Rita unwittingly set herself up for failure, and we cannot caution you enough against making this mistake. Rita's crackers and peanut butter were, from the start, a test, which she predicted she would flunk. She bought the goodies to prove how bad she really is and how incorrigible a habit she has. She was never able to convince herself that these forbidden foods were in her house to stay.

It takes determination, courage, and patience to see yourself through the initial step of legalizing food. You will test yourself the way children test their parents until you're certain that you mean it when you say that ice cream is no different from lettuce. But if you stay with it, eventually no food will feel dangerous, and all foods will become your friends for life.

On the Aisle: As you enter your local supermarket armed with your list of wishes, get ready for adventure. Our advice is to head for the aisles and have fun. You are convinced that you have a right to eat what you want. Indeed, you recognize that only by eating what you want do you stand a chance of getting beyond your eating problems.

For many compulsive eaters, however, a trip to the supermarket is a frightening experience. "How can I go into my local supermarket where everyone knows me and start filling my cart with huge quantities of food?" Helen asked.

"Everyone will think I'm crazy," Sid agreed. "They'll look at my cart and think, 'No wonder he looks the way he does.'"

"If I had a cart filled with everything I want in surplus, I don't think I could look the checkout clerk in the eye," Irene concluded.

We understand these fears. They are not unfounded. If you are fat and fill your shopping cart with forbidden foods, you will undoubtedly get some judgmental looks. The truth is that you have given yourself those very same looks and been harder than anyone else on yourself. Now is the time, however, for you to be kind to yourself. You need to make this first shopping expedition as pleasant an experience as you can and do whatever is necessary so that other people's reactions don't get in your way.

Some of the people with whom we work make it a point of shopping somewhere other than their usual supermarket until they feel more comfortable with the contents of their cart. "It's worth the extra few blocks' walk to me," one person said, "to be in a place where everyone doesn't know me. It's been two weeks since I've legalized foods," she went on, "and I think I'm beginning to feel more comfortable with the whole thing now."

At one workshop someone suggested announcing at the checkout counter that you are giving a dinner party, although many in the group felt that for them such an announcement was an old compulsive-eating trick and they preferred not to make any excuses. Someone else said that it was helpful for her to phone in her first few orders and have them delivered.

However you deal with your initial discomfort, the critical thing is to recognize that you have a right to eat what you want. Indeed, the only way you can finally resolve your addiction to food is to eat what you want without sneaking it. No matter what other people think or say, you are headed on a new course that requires no explanation unless you wish to give⁂ it—which brings us to your family and friends.

Home Again, Home Again . . .

Not too long after you asked your kids to hide their Halloween candy because you found it too tempting, you arrive home with three bags of Milky Ways. "Hey, Mom," your nine-year-old says, "I thought you didn't want to be fat."

Your husband walks into the kitchen and finds you eating a peanut butter and fluff sandwich. "What's up, honey?" he asks. "You spent months starving yourself. Do you want to undo all your hard work?"

Your family loves you. They care about your well-being, and they say these things out of their concern for you. They have listened to you for years, and they've learned their lessons well. You have enlisted their help with regard to your weight. They know, better than anyone, how much you hate your body. They have watched you run the paces of the diet race over the years. And they've heard you scold yourself during the binge cycle. It makes perfect sense for your family to cheer you on as you play Change Your Shape and Change Your Life. They do, after all, have your best interests at heart. They, like you, are concerned that your weight will skyrocket if you don't exercise restraint.

How do you enlist their support as you attempt to learn, for the first time, to feed yourself? For starters, you'll need to reeducate them as you reeducate yourself. Before you bring the food into your house, you have to prepare your family.

One woman did it this way. She said, "I know that I have counted on you to help me resist certain foods, but I now see that trying to resist food only makes me want it more. I want to get over my fear of food and learn to eat in a less driven way. It may seem crazy to you, but I've decided to lift all my food bans. I'm not sure what will happen, but I've got to break away from all the dieting I've always done. I still need your help and support but in a different way. This time I need you to stop monitoring me. I know that what I'm about to do will seem bizarre and probably upset you. All I ask is that you try to understand. It won't be easy for you not to comment, but if you slip, I'll remind you."

It will probably help if you ask family members to read this book. It will probably be as hard for them to accept our ideas as it was for you, however, so don't be surprised or annoyed if they don't offer you a lot of support initially. Keep in mind that, in a sense, you are separating yourself from them. After years of looking to others for rules and guidance regarding what you eat, you are announcing that you plan to go it alone. The people closest to you are likely to feel rejected before they can move on to a new kind of support.

Plunging ahead without the help and support of your family may be hard on you. "In the beginning my husband was furious," Anna told her group. "He kept telling me that I was setting a terrible example for our kids. That really got me where it hurt." After a while Anna came to believe in her heart of hearts that her new approach to food and eating was a very good example for her children. She was teaching them to be unafraid of foods, to use food to feed physiological rather than emotional hunger. Until you feel entirely secure about what you're doing, however, it's a good idea to try to avoid confrontations. It's also useful to look for ways to reassure family members that they need not lose out because you are meeting your own needs. Some people we've known have found ways to make this clear.

Arlene, a forty-two-year-old mother of three, got everyone in her family to make a list of foods they wanted. Her next shopping trip was exciting, and especially satisfying, for everyone. It didn't take long for everyone in her family to grow accustomed to having what they liked on hand.

The Cupboards

It's important, in a household where everyone has his special foods, to respect the fact that certain foods are earmarked for certain people. If, for example, Anna bought herself some sweet potatoes, she should be able to count on having them there when she wants them. If she reaches for them and discovers that her daughter ate them, the benefit of stocking up will have been lost.

It's crucial to know that your favorite cheese, bread, yogurt, candy, cake, whatever, won't be snatched by anyone else. This program requires your being able to count on having enough of what you want when you want it so that you can begin to relax around food. If you're worried about who's getting to the goodies first, you'll be as anxious as ever and find yourself eating because you're afraid they'll disappear rather than because you're hungry.

We suggest that you have a shelf in the refrigerator and cupboard marked with your name. Alternatively, put your name on any food item that you wish to legalize and tell your family that you do not want them to eat from your supply. Tell those who may be tempted by the foods on your shelf that they can fill their own shelves with the very same food. They cannot, however, eat your supply, because if they do, you won't have it when you need it. After a while everyone will learn that securing special foods has to do with tending to your own needs rather than depriving other people. Although at first it may seem antithetical to the spirit of family sharing, you will all discover that you cannot really begin to share until you are confident that what you have is yours.

"At first everyone was furious when I put my name on six chocolate bars," Irene said. "My husband said, 'You don't need six of these. That's plenty for all of us.' I could understand where he was coming from, but I didn't buckle under. In fact, I felt very angry. The point is that *he* was telling me what was enough for me. I need to find that out for myself, and I can't find it out unless I have *more* than I need. I asked him how much chocolate he wanted and then asked my kids. I put on my coat that moment and went out and bought a dozen Hershey bars for each member of the family, and I made a rule right then that whatever was in a personal cupboard could not be eaten without the owner's permission."

"I had a similar experience," said Herb. "But I put four blank pieces of paper up on the fridge and wrote names at the top of each—one for each of my kids, one for my wife, and one for me. I instituted a plan whereby each of us writes down what we want during the week and on Saturday, when we do our big family shopping, we gather the lists. It's really worked out well for us."

There are lots of different ways to make sure that everyone's appetite is tended to. It's important to keep in mind, however, that the goal is to bring in as many of your favorite foods as possible and to have access to them when you want them.

Legal Costs

By now, most of you have begun to wonder about the cost of legalizing foods. It's one thing to talk about buying thick lamb chops, but quite another to reach into your purse and come up with the money. "Sure I'd like to buy everything I want," one man commented. "I'd like to buy all the food I want just as I'd like to buy all the clothing and all the stereo equipment I want. But the reality is that I don't have all the *money* I want."

All of our lives are circumscribed by what we can and cannot afford, and the process of legalizing food does sound very expensive. We can only say that the outlay of money is greatest when you start and that the returns make the expense worthwhile. It is, in a sense, an investment. We are accustomed to investing in things like a good education, which benefits us in the long run. If we don't invest, we pay by diminishing the rest of our lives.

Sue told us that she was amazed by how much money she spent the first month of legalizing. "I really bought everything I wanted and lots of it. After three months of doing this, I've noticed that the cost is coming down. I prefer the more expensive brands of certain foods, but I no longer have to buy as much as I did at first. For one thing, I'm eating less, and for another, I no longer have to prove to myself that I can buy whatever I need. If I want something and don't have it, I just go and get it without doing a number on myself."

Legalizing foods is, in a sense, like embarking on a new business venture. If you were to open a shop, you would initially lay out a great deal of capital on stock. During the first several months of business you would learn which stock sells and which doesn't. By the time you were ready to reorder you would know a great deal more about what and how much to buy. Your second order would be based on the demand of your clientele.

The same holds true for the start-up phase of food legalization. Once you know what you want and need to have around, you won't always have to restock in quite the same way. Very few of us have unlimited amounts of money to spend, and we all have to work within the confines of our budgets. Keep in mind, however, that when you get the hang of living with surplus you won't always require the same quantity to prove to yourself that you can provide what you want when you want it.

The issue of buying in excess also raises the question of the inevitable waste that occurs when you begin to legalize foods. If you buy more fresh bread than you can eat, some of that bread will probably get stale or moldy. Although none of us feels good about wasting food, we know that finishing the food on our plate has no direct impact on the issue of world hunger and that the food we throw out would not have been sent to Biafra. However, if we eat it when we are not hungry, it is also wasted.

Once you get to know yourself as an eater, you will be in a better position to judge how much you need to buy, and you will waste less food. The start-up costs and waste of legalizing are necessary to help you overcome what is probably the central problem of your life—your addictive relationship to food.

If you think about the pain you've suffered over the years as a result of your compulsive eating and add up the money you've spent on diets, diet books, and "cures"—not to mention binges—you'll find that, in the long run, it's easier and cheaper to take care of your appetite than to fight it.

The Plan
Phase 2

Feeding Yourself

– 9 –

Food on Demand

Legalizing food and living comfortably in the present are the first, crucial steps you must take toward resolving your compulsive eating problem. Only when you feel free in a world of food can you tackle the major question that confronts any compulsive eater, namely, how to eat.

In the chapters that follow, we will reacquaint you with a way of eating that you once knew but long ago forgot—food on demand, which we believe is the antidote for compulsive eating. These chapters will help you answer the three questions that constitute the "how to" of eating: When should you eat? What should you eat? How much should you eat?

Our position on change has been that it flows from acceptance and knowledge. Needless to say, we believe that you won't be able to change the way you currently eat until you understand and accept it. How *do* you eat? Let's take a look.

The Urge to Eat

Ask anyone why we need food and they'll tell you, "It's simple. We have to eat or else we'd die." Food is our fuel. It keeps us going. For the compulsive eater, however, food fulfills this function only incidentally. The "hungry" signal is rarely what sends compulsive eaters to food. More often a compulsive eater eats in response to anxiety. Therefore, we find it useful to think in terms of two kinds of hunger: stomach hunger and mouth hunger.

Stomach Hunger: Stomach hunger—by which we mean *physiological* hunger—is connected to our physiological need to refuel. It's the kind of hunger that sustains life. Compulsive eaters rarely experience stomach hunger. Indeed, compulsive eating is, by definition, eating that serves functions other than the satisfaction of physiological hunger.

Mouth Hunger: Compulsive eaters most often eat from mouth hunger. Mouth hunger—or *psychological* hunger—has nothing to do with the sustenance of life. It includes the eating you do "just because it's there," "because you have to put something in your mouth," "because it tastes good," "because it looks so delicious," "because it's time for breakfast/lunch/dinner," "because someone went to the trouble to prepare it," "because it would be a shame to throw it away," "because you feel lonely/anxious/depressed," or "because you feel happy/excited/like celebrating." Mouth hunger is what summons you to the refrigerator as soon as you sit down to work. And mouth hunger is what compels you to hit the road at 11:30 P.M. in search of an all-night ice cream stand. Finally, mouth hunger is what continues to send spoon after spoon of ice cream to your mouth long after you've begun to feel ill.

Until now you've had a mild awareness of the difference between mouth hunger and stomach hunger. Mouth hunger is the kind you've attempted to control with diets. Until recently, you've responded to it by chastising yourself. "What's wrong with me," you've said. "Those cookies were the last thing I needed. I have no control. Why did I do it?"

It is essential that you learn to recognize the difference between mouth hunger and stomach hunger and to recognize, rather than judge, which kind is operating when you have the urge to eat.

The Ledger

If you were to create a ledger with two columns, one labeled MOUTH HUNGER and the other STOMACH HUNGER and observe your eating habits over the course of the next few days, the chances are that, if you're a compulsive eater, you'd have many checks in the mouth hunger column and very few in the one labeled stomach hunger.

You might want to make such a ledger to keep track of when you're eating from stomach hunger and when from mouth hunger in order to become acquainted with your present eating patterns. It's important to understand, however, that this ledger will be helpful to you only if you can keep track of your manner of eating without judging it, in much the same way as we recommended you learn to look at your body in a mirror.

It sometimes helps in creating a healthy, nonjudgmental stance to regard yourself as an anthropologist observing the eating habits of someone in a foreign culture. The eating you observe, of course, will be your own. Each time you eat or think about food, ask yourself, "Why do I want to eat right now? Am I hungry? Or is something else prompting my desire for food?" You'll need to remind yourself over and over again that it is your job to notice and collect data, not to judge or intervene. If you discover that keeping a ledger promotes the old diet mentality, if you castigate yourself and try to stop yourself from eating every time you put a check in the mouth hunger column, abandon the ledger in favor of mental notes.

Once you have developed an overview of your eating, you are in a position to do something about it. First, you'll need to define the problem. If you're a compulsive eater, and if you've been able to maintain distance while keeping a ledger, you can, quite literally, see your problem on the page before you. You can look at your ledger and see that the vast majority of your checks fall under the heading of mouth hunger.

The checks in that column reflect the reality that, more often than not, feelings other than stomach hunger take you to food. You reach for food rather than attempt to name your problem and think it through when you feel anxious or uneasy. You use food as first aid. You fall down, scrape your knee, and run to the freezer for a dish of ice cream.

There are, of course, many reasons why you attempt to heal yourself with food, and we'll address them later. What's most important now, however, is that after years of using food to heal your wounds, you have forgotten that it has another function. You have forgotten what stomach hunger is all about.

The Hunger Connection

To cure your compulsive eating problem you must reestablish the connection between food and stomach hunger. To become a noncompulsive or "normal" eater, you must act like a normal eater and put food back where it belongs. Essentially, you must shift the checks in your ledger from the mouth hunger column to the stomach hunger one.

Moving the checks from one column to the other is not as easy as it sounds. Remember that your need to eat in a driven way has endured despite a history of attempts to extinguish it. Eating from mouth hunger has been a trusted companion over the years, calming you when nothing else could. Don't expect to say "From now on I'm only going to eat from stomach hunger" and simply be able to do it. Such a declaration reflects a wish or a fantasy, but it has nothing to do with your needs. If you could put a stop to your compulsive eating by wishing it weren't so, you would have done it long ago.

We do not think that you should stop eating because of mouth hunger. We have something different in mind. Our goal is to help you eliminate the experience of mouth hunger entirely, that is, to stop turning to food unless you're hungry. The difference between controlling and eliminating mouth hunger is critical. It is the difference between eating compulsively and eating normally, between controlling your eating and curing it.

We do not want you to wrench yourself away from the refrigerator door. We want you to eat from mouth hunger for as long as you *feel* mouth hunger. We simply want you to look forward to the day when you will no longer experience it.

Demand Feeding—For Adults

You are going to eat your way out of your eating problem by putting food back where it belongs. Each time you feed yourself when your stomach is hungry, you are accomplishing two important tasks—nourishing yourself physiologically and nurturing yourself emotionally. You are repeating an event which, from infancy on, has symbolized trust. Indeed, feeding yourself appropriately satisfies two most basic human needs, those of physical and emotional sustenance.

Our cure for compulsive eating requires that you return to the beginning of your life vis-à-vis eating and start all over again. We call this approach, based on the premise that each of us is born knowing how to eat in a normal, noncompulsive way, demand feeding for adults.

All infants know how to eat when they're hungry and stop

eating when they're full. Secure infants have learned, through endless sequences of feeling hungry and being fed, that the world responds reliably to their needs. Through a long and complicated process of development, infants who have learned to count on the people who care for them come to learn that they can count on themselves as well. Infants who are fed whenever they cry for food come to regard themselves as effective. Indeed, each time a hungry infant cries for food and is fed, the message that her needs can be met is reinforced, and consequently she becomes a bit stronger psychologically.

Unfortunately, somewhere along the line between infancy and adulthood, your ability to recognize and feed your stomach hunger was overcome by your compulsion to eat. Many of you have probably wondered how this happened. Let us dispel a few misconceptions.

There is no single cause for your compulsive eating; it is complex. People do not become compulsive eaters because their mothers dropped them on their head or because they were fed on a schedule rather than on demand. Many people become compulsive eaters because they respond to the dictates of the culture and start dieting. Others begin to eat compulsively when they are unable to master a new stage in development or when they are in considerable conflict. They reach out for food as a symbol of an earlier sense of security just as someone else might talk a lot or clean the house or spend money or exercise. Our predilections for certain modes of tension release stem from our innate constitution, our family style, and our upbringing.

Whatever its genesis, compulsive eating always involves the separation of food from stomach hunger. The fact that so many of you are out of touch with this most primitive experience of feeding stomach hunger is terribly sad. It means, essentially, that you have lost your most basic guideline for existence. You no longer know when to reach out for supplies. Life without this basic survival mechanism is, to say the least, disequilibrating, but take heart. The situation is not hopeless.

Your ability to recognize and feed your stomach hunger was only submerged, not destroyed by, your compulsion to eat. Each of you still has an internal mechanism that will tell you when your stomach is empty and when it is full. Once you get back in touch with that mechanism, you will be able to respond to it.

Your first order of business is to put yourself back on a demand-feeding schedule. You must allow yourself to get hungry and eat on your own schedule, just as infants get hungry and eat on theirs. One day you may eat twice, another day six times, another day eight times, and so on. All that matters is that you eat according to your hunger rather than to the clock. If you're hungry at four you need to eat at four, even if "dinner" won't be served until six. Waiting those extra two hours puts you out of touch with your hunger. Your goal, for the moment, is to abandon entirely all external cues like calorie charts, mealtimes, or social gatherings so you can rediscover the internal cues you buried years ago. Your body will direct the process.

Each time you experience physiological hunger and respond to it by feeding yourself, you learn that you can care for yourself effectively, that you can meet your own needs, and that your needs are worthy of attention. This message is so powerful that the more often you experience it, the stronger your psychological base will be and the better you'll feel. Consequently, the more times you eat from stomach hunger every day, the better. Ironically, the resolution of your addiction to food lies in a reawakening of the very experience you have spent the better part of your life attempting to extinguish. You have tried time and again to get around your hunger and *not* to eat. Now, the time has come for you to do an about-face and eat from stomach hunger as often as possible.

It's not too late to start over. The twofold task is to learn to recognize stomach hunger and to start responding to it.

Recognizing Stomach Hunger

Simple as it sounds, the question "Are you hungry?" is a profound one for compulsive eaters, for hunger is generally the last thing they think about when they reach for food. Most compulsive eaters tell us that by the time they reach adulthood they are either entirely out of touch with the feeling of stomach hunger or that the signal is very dim.

The whole notion of eating in response to stomach hunger is so alien to compulsive eaters that they are shocked when they hear a noncompulsive eater turn down the offer of a meal with "Thanks, but I'm not hungry right now." What, they wonder, does hunger have to do with anything? The more out of touch you are with the connection between stomach hunger and eating, the more checks you have in the mouth hunger column of your ledger, the less likely you are to have reaped the psychological benefits that come from being your own feeder.

When the Signal Is Dim: If you are among those compulsive eaters who *do* experience stomach hunger but for whom the signal is dim, we recommend that you start making a conscious effort to tune in to your hunger. As long as you are eating from mouth hunger, of course, the signals for stomach hunger will be few and far between. Your stomach cannot tell you it's hungry if your mouth has just filled it to take care of some other feeling. The more you look forward to the experience of stomach hunger, however, the more apt you are to find it.

Looking forward to eating from stomach hunger starts the checks moving from the mouth hunger to the stomach hunger side of the ledger. If you are eager to find occasions to eat out of stomach hunger, you will sometimes be able to overlook the urgings of mouth hunger.

When the Signal Is Gone: Unfortunately, many compulsive eaters have absolutely no memory of stomach hunger or the satisfaction that comes from feeding it. We've discovered, in the course of our work with such people, that they often find the idea of stomach hunger genuinely frightening. There are several possible reasons for their fear.

The feeling of stomach hunger is a reminder of bad times for people who have experienced real deprivation in their lives. They cannot feel hungry without recalling all the other emotions that accompanied hunger in their memories. The children of such people usually have a related fear—each time they were pushed to eat as children, their parents' concern about potential famine was driven home to them, and they fear that the feeling of hunger will lead to disaster.

Some compulsive eaters fear the intensity of hunger. They fear that so strong a feeling will overwhelm them or cause them to feel out of control. What if their hunger cannot be satisfied? What if, once they start eating, they cannot stop?

Finally, many compulsive eaters will not allow themselves to feel hunger because they resent having to rely on themselves for nurturance. The primitive feeling of stomach hunger reminds them of early needs that went unmet. They are angry about what they didn't get from others long ago. Indeed, their anger at having to be their own feeder interferes with the pleasure they might otherwise feel at the realization that they can, at long last, care for themselves in an appropriately tender way.

Interestingly, people are not always aware that they are

afraid to feel hungry. They make the discovery only when they are confronted by their inability to put off eating long enough for the sensation to appear.

If you are among those who fear the experience of stomach hunger, you must bring your fear into the open and look at it objectively. Realistically, physiological hunger is a sensation that is quite easily taken care of with the appropriate amount of food. The fear you attach to feeling stomach hunger is a remnant of your childhood concerns about neediness. You must reassure yourself that you are ready, willing, and able to nurture yourself. As a matter of fact, all compulsive eaters need to welcome stomach hunger by reassuring themselves that they can and will provide themselves with all the food they need, whenever they need it.

Of course, your years of self-deprivation, of dieting and self-contempt, have given you precisely the opposite message. Compulsive eaters have no basis on which to trust their ability as feeders. Not having nurtured themselves in the past, they have no reason to believe that they will do so in the future. In the past, they've shouted, insisted on abstinence, curtailed the pleasure they might have had from food, and, most certainly, never taken the trouble to ask themselves "Am I hungry?"

The first step in coming to terms with a history of uncaring behavior involves a complete about-face. You can overcome the insecurity you feel about yourself as a nurturer by providing food in great quantity and by putting an end, once and for all, to your self-contemptuous scolding.

If you are a compulsive eater who no longer knows what stomach hunger feels like, we suggest that you start talking about it with your friends. Ask them to describe what they mean when they say "I'm hungry." You'll find that different people experience hunger in different ways at different times. Some describe an empty feeling in the pit of their stomach; others talk of a slight sense of nausea; still others mention a feeling in the back of the throat.

There's a difference, of course, between feeling hungry and letting yourself get too hungry. When we talk about feeding yourself on demand, we are referring to your initial signal of hunger. The first step in self-demand feeding is to respond to your hunger with enthusiasm. "Oh, terrific, I'm hungry. That means it's time to eat!"

Responding to Stomach Hunger

Now that you've discovered stomach hunger, what do you do with it? The answer is quite simple—you feed it. You feed yourself when and as often as you feel hungry. We live in a culture that is more oriented toward preventing hunger than responding to it. "I'd better eat now in case I get hungry later" is more the norm than "Great, I'm hungry. I'm going to get something to eat." Keep in mind, as you begin to focus on the feeling of stomach hunger, that you are trying to move the checks in your ledger from the mouth hunger to the stomach hunger column. It's good to get hungry often. The more often you eat when you're hungry, the faster the checks in your ledger will shift.

The relationship between stomach and mouth hunger is converse. The more you eat from stomach hunger, the less you will want to eat from mouth hunger. The most obvious reason is that when you eat often from stomach hunger your desire to eat is well satisfied. There is, however, a much more profound explanation for why the checks move as they do from the mouth to the stomach hunger column.

Learning to eat from stomach hunger after many years of eating from mouth hunger is not simply a change of habit, nor is it a mere reconditioning of your eating behavior. Each time you feed yourself when you are hungry, you demonstrate to yourself that you can respond to your needs. Think of it this way: as you become more attuned to yourself you will feel more secure. After all, you are becoming an excellent self-nurturer. You have learned to feed yourself when you're hungry and deal with yourself sympathetically when you need to resort to food for reasons other than hunger. The knowledge that you can turn to someone so caring and tender as yourself makes it less likely that you'll need to turn to food when you're in trouble.

Nina had been trying to feed herself on demand for several months and told us she was anxious about an upcoming visit to her parents. "Usually," she said, "as soon as I walk in the door I go to my mom's refrigerator and proceed to eat my way through the visit. I'm not aware of being unhappy while I'm there, but the memories must be what get me going. I've spent most of my life on one diet or another, and the struggles about food in that house were constant."

This visit, however, was different for Nina. As in the past, she *did* walk into her parents' house and check out the refrigerator. For the first time in her life, however, her parents' full fridge didn't look much different from hers because Nina no longer kept her own refrigerator bare to avoid temptation. This was a reassuring discovery. Nina did note, with some distress, that while she had been hungry when they sat down to dinner, she had eaten far too much, and that during the drive home she had eaten all the leftovers her mother had packed for her. She was upset about it, but pleased that, on the whole, she had been less driven to eat during this visit with her family than she had ever been in the past. This realization left her feeling optimistic about her future.

If you think of Nina's experience with eating on demand as an attempt to reparent herself, you will see that her optimism is well founded. From that perspective her trip home looks like this: Before Nina visited her parents she had been feeding herself on demand for two weeks. During that time, let's assume, she had had many experiences of eating from stomach hunger and had demonstrated to herself many times that she could reliably meet her own needs. Although Nina enjoys seeing her parents, her visits to them also make her tense. Perhaps she has fears about being too dependent on them. Maybe the ghosts of diets-past that linger in her parents' house are too painful.

Whatever causes Nina's tension is significant, and eventually she will want to understand exactly what it is. We do not believe, however, that compulsive eaters must understand all their conflicts in order to resolve their addiction to food. Nina doesn't need to unearth the source of her tension at the moment. All she has to do to resolve her compulsive eating is to continue to eat from stomach hunger as often as possible.

When Nina again visits her parents in two weeks, she will have had that additional time to reinforce her own responsive "parenting." It's reasonable to assume that by then Nina will have eaten out of stomach hunger two or three times more than she had at her previous visit. Her increasing number of experiences of eating from stomach hunger will have had a cumulative effect on Nina, and she will be different as a result of them.

We are not suggesting that by her second visit Nina will have resolved all her problems. Indeed, she may not seem very different to you, to us, or even to herself. But because she has been feeding herself and talking to herself about her eating and her weight in a sympathetic, not an abusive way, Nina will feel differently about herself.

When she arrives at her parents' house Nina may not feel the same desperate need to eat that she did in the past. At some point, either on this visit or later, she will be able to stop eating dinner as soon as her hunger has been satisfied, and she won't have to gobble up the leftovers on the way home. There will come a time when Nina can visit her parents and eat what she's hungry for and not from anxiety. When that happens, Nina will probably feel comfortable enough to know what she's feeling and begin to think about what's causing her anxiety.

Impossible? Not at all. Nina's progress is not only possible, it's probable. But Nina, and those like her, have to give themselves a nudge in the right direction.

The Nudge: When you embark on demand feeding, most of the checks in your ledger are in the mouth hunger column, with very few on the side of stomach hunger. You are now going to *nudge* yourself in the direction of stomach hunger.

Each time you want to eat, you ask yourself "Am I hungry?" If the answer is yes, you say "Great. This is an opportunity to feed myself on demand." Each time you respond to hunger with food you are reinforcing a connection that came asunder at some point in your past. It takes many such experiences to revive this basic link between hunger and eating, but it must be done. This link, after all, is central to life.

But what happens when the answer to "Am I hungry?" is "No, I just want to eat!" Rest assured, there will be times when you still want to eat from mouth hunger. At such times, we suggest the following internal dialogue:

FEEDER: Would you like to try to wait until you're hungry? Remember, you're starting to eat out of stomach hunger and if you eat now from mouth hunger, you'll be throwing your stomach hunger schedule off.

EATER: No, I don't want to wait. I want to eat.

FEEDER: Fine. What exactly does your mouth want to eat? Remember, if your stomach isn't hungry you don't have to think about filling it up. All you have to think about is putting exactly what you want into your mouth.

EATER: I want a hot fudge sundae.

FEEDER: Fine. Let's get it. By the way, I'm sorry that something is making you so anxious that food is the only thing that will calm you down. Remember, don't berate yourself after you've eaten and maybe later you'll be able to figure out what's bothering you and perhaps find stomach hunger again.

The Binge

As you begin to feed yourself on demand, you can expect your progress to be uneven. Most people learn fairly quickly to be kind to themselves, to allow themselves lapses, and to expect that, on occasion, they will eat from mouth hunger. They also learn that if they don't yell at themselves when they have such lapses, they eat less during them.

When a compulsive eater who is on his way to becoming a noncompulsive eater finds himself binging, however, he tends to forget what he's learned and to panic. The greater his panic, the more probable it is that he will try to scream himself out of the binge in a voice filled with anger. "Can't you get a grip on yourself? Your eating is _really_ out of control. You're making yourself sick. You just have to stop."

Think back to your last binge. Did yelling at yourself help you to stop? It undoubtedly just prolonged the binge. Attempting to stop a binge by screaming at yourself is like attempting to stop a skid by slamming on your brakes. Every experienced driver knows that when you're spinning on ice and hit your brakes, your car's inertia intensifies the skid; but if you attempt to go with the skid, the car will eventually stop itself.

That's the way it is with a binge. If you fight it with angry, abusive words, you only prolong it. If, on the other hand, you go with the binge, it will come to its own end. What does "going with the binge" involve?

- No more abusive remarks. If you find yourself yelling, remind yourself that negative thoughts make you feel bad, and feeling bad makes you want to binge.
- Replace your yelling with a reminder that your binge is a symptom of anxiety. Something is making you uncomfortable and you need soothing. You need compassion, not rebuke.
- Tell yourself that you don't have to know *why* you're upset before you can be sympathetic to yourself.
- Be as tender and nurturing to yourself during your binge as you possibly can. Give yourself the foods you really want.
- Go back to the beginning of this new approach to eating and make sure to have food available in large quantities, to wear comfortable clothing that you like; and to stay off the scale.

Remember, all binges come to an end. All you have to do is coast and gently begin to nudge yourself back in the direction of stomach hunger.

Ellen knew that a binge was on the horizon because when she entered her house she headed straight for the cupboard, where the first thing she saw was a box of saltine crackers and a jar of jam, her old binge standbys. But when she grabbed for the crackers and jam she took the trouble to think. "I really don't even like saltines," she told herself. "They're my old binge food. If I'm going to binge now, at least I should eat something I really love. Why compromise?"

Ellen didn't panic. Instead, she went to the freezer, took

out her newly legalized mint Oreo cookie ice cream, and went to town. Later she told us, "You know, it does make a difference when you treat yourself well during a binge. I've noticed that if I give myself my favorite food, rather than punish myself with second-rate food, I end up eating less and my binge doesn't last as long." Ellen discovered that self-care is a good deal more productive than self-criticism.

Stephen made a similar discovery. "I had a bad binge the other night," he explained, "and I woke up in the morning furious with myself. I remembered that trashing myself would only make things worse. So I decided not to scream at myself for feeling desperate. Instead, I forced myself to put on the new suit I bought last week. I continued to eat out of mouth hunger that day, but I was more relaxed about it. By late evening I was finally able to feel stomach hunger again. And let me tell you, it felt *good*. It's really true that when you know you're not going to yell at yourself for binging, you don't eat nearly as much."

* * *

We've said that the cure for compulsive eating requires feeding yourself on demand, that is, eating when you're hungry. But eating is a bit more complicated than that. Not only do you need to know when to eat, but you also need to know what and how much to eat. When, what, and how much are the subjects of the next three chapters.

- 10 -

When to Eat

When? What? How much? The answers to these questions form the core of every diet, but now that you've abandoned diets, you're on your own. It should come as no surprise that we, having emphasized the importance of getting in touch with your individual hunger patterns, have no intention of answering these questions for you. We don't think you have to turn to an outside authority—a diet, social convention, or the sight and smell of something tempting—for advice on when to eat, what to eat, and when you've had enough. Indeed, we think that you already have the answers.

You don't yet have much experience eating in response to internal cues, but the cues are there, and they are deserving of respect. You probably know a lot about yourself as a worker, spouse, lover, friend, parent, sibling, and so on. As a recent ex-dieter, however, you know very little about who you are as an eater. Now is the time to find out, and the place to start is with the question "When?"

When Do I Eat?

The time to eat is when you're hungry. Lest that answer seem simplistic, we must remind you that getting in touch with stomach hunger has been no small task. Most of your eating so far has been in response to mouth hunger. You've reached for food automatically, without thinking about whether your impulse to eat had anything to do with an empty stomach. Once you begin to recognize the signals of stomach hunger you can do yourself no greater favor than trying to respond to them by eating when you're hungry.

If you can respond to your stomach rather than the clock, you'll soon discover that there are no set rules governing appetite. You have your own internal clock, which regulates your hunger schedule. Some of you, for example, may not be hungry first thing in the morning even though your parents, and their parents before them, stressed the importance of a hearty breakfast. Others may need steak, eggs, and home fries before they can think straight. Some of you may crave food before bedtime, while others discover that late-night eating interferes with sleep. Many of you may discover that your hunger patterns vary each day, and some of you will find that your patterns run a particular course and then change slowly over time. The important thing to understand is that your hunger, like your signature, is unique.

The Meaninglessness of Meals

Eating when you are hungry means abandoning all standard notions of "the right time to eat." Most of our eating is more oriented to the clock on the wall than to our internal time clock. Only after you've abandoned the habit of three meals a day or business drinks at five or dinner at six can you begin to think about when you really need to eat.

Of course it's difficult for people who have been raised on breakfast, lunch, and dinner to suddenly begin eating when they're hungry and not eating when they're not. It may be necessary, as you begin to eat when you're hungry, to eliminate the words *breakfast, lunch,* and *dinner* from your vocabulary. We find it helpful, at the start, to think in terms of eating experiences rather than meals.

Many people respond with great sadness to our suggestion that they abandon traditional mealtimes, and no wonder. Many of them have in the past given up the pleasure of mealtime to eat cabbage and grapefruit with no good, long-term results. When we tell them to give up traditional meals, they fear that they will never again be able to sit down to breakfast with family or meet friends for dinner at a favorite restaurant. We are pleased to report that such fear is unfounded.

There will come a time when you find a comfortable place for yourself within the framework of traditional mealtimes, even if you don't eat during them. Socially enforced feeding schedules are an obstacle when you are beginning to hook into your own inner time clock. Once you are more experienced at eating when you're hungry, you will be able to adjust your hunger to meet a particular time or event. At the start, however, you have to make the task at hand as easy as possible for yourself. To that end, the following exercise will prove useful.

An Eating Exercise

The goal of this exercise is to get hungry as often as possible during the course of a day. We suggest that you choose a day when you feel most in control of your life, one on which you are relatively relaxed. For some people the weekend, away from the stress of work routines, is best. Others are more comfortable approaching this exercise during the week, when work schedules give structure to their time. Whichever day you pick for the experiment, you'll have to give up all routine eating in favor of feeling your body's signals, and you must assure yourself access to an ample supply of food.

It's helpful, as you embark on this exercise, to eat only small amounts each time you feel hungry. We will later discuss how to know what amount of food correctly matches your hunger signal. For the purpose of this exercise, however, we would like you to limit your quantities to ensure as many hunger experiences as possible. If you eat a small amount of food, it won't be too long before you feel hungry again.

Greet the day you've chosen for this exercise by checking in with your stomach before you get out of bed. When you wake, give yourself a few quiet moments in bed and think about whether or not you feel hungry. If your stomach is not signaling hunger, allow yourself time to shower, dress, and go about your early morning business. Half an hour later, sit down and give yourself another quiet moment to tune in to your stomach. Are you hungry yet?

If the answer is yes—if you feel an emptiness in your stomach—have something to eat. If you are still not hungry, pass up the breakfast you routinely eat and proceed with your day. As you do, you might think about how often you eat breakfast when you aren't hungry, how often your hand reaches for the cereal bowl because you think you won't have time for it later when you're hungry. We call the eating that you do to prevent hunger "prophylactic eating," eating that keeps you in a constant state of fullness and obscures the signals of stomach hunger that originate from within.

Continue to check in with your stomach throughout the day. "Am I hungry?" is the key question. As soon as you respond with a yes, it's time to eat. If, for example, you get an empty feeling in your stomach at 11:00 A.M., it means you should eat at 11:01. Your task requires that you respond to your hunger immediately rather than waiting another hour until lunchtime. Take the time at eleven, stop what you're doing, and eat something. When you've finished, you can proceed with your day.

We said at the onset that the goal for this day is to experience hunger as often as possible. By the time you go to bed at night you should have a real sense of what hunger feels like. Review the day. Think about how often you were hungry. Think about each time you ate and how you felt when you were through. Take the time to notice how it felt to eat with stomach hunger. Ask yourself how that feeling was different from the one you have when you eat from mouth hunger. Most people are surprised by how much more pleasurable eating is when their stomachs really ask for it. That pleasure makes them look forward to more such experiences and encourages them to see this exercise not as an isolated event but as an example of what life can and should be like when you feed yourself on demand.

To ensure the success of this exercise and of demand feeding, you will need an ample supply of food at all times. Which brings us to the "food bag."

The Food Bag

"Oh, I got hungry at work around three o'clock but I had to wait until six, when I got home, to get something to eat." "I only had a cup of coffee for breakfast and didn't get hungry until eleven. By that time I figured I only had an hour and a half until lunch, so I held off."

If you're going to prove to yourself that you can meet your own needs in a tender, caring way, you must have food with you at all times to avoid such situations. Holding off for an hour or two is the ultimate in desertion for the compulsive eater who is attempting to feed stomach hunger. The only way to be sure you have food to eat as soon as you feel hungry is to carry it with you.

What to Pack: As you become more experienced at feeding yourself, you'll develop a good sense of how to match your hunger with the specific food you want to eat. The more refined this sense becomes, the easier it will be for you to anticipate your needs and pack your food bag. Until then, we suggest that you carry an ample assortment of foods with you at all times.

This doesn't require packing a cooler every time you step out. It simply means taking a few of the foods you think you will be hungry for. If you've just legalized certain foods you can be certain that they will be what you crave: pistachio nuts, M & M's, cookies, fruit, cheese. Think about what you like and be certain to keep it within reach.

Remember, these "carry" foods are not snack foods. Once you dispense with the idea of breakfast, lunch, and dinner, you also dispense with the idea of between-meal snacks. The things you pack in your bag are simply foods to be eaten whenever your stomach is empty.

You can carry them in your purse, briefcase, coat pocket, knapsack, or a paper bag. We've often thought it would be a good idea to have a tote bag with FOOD printed on it. Desk drawers, office refrigerators, and gym lockers are all fine cupboards-away-from-home. The specific foods to carry will vary from person to person. The key, however, is to have what you want when you want it.

The Feelings You Carry with the Bag: Many people resist the notion of carrying food around with them. "It's too messy," one man said. "I wouldn't know what to bring," said another. "Things will go bad." "I can always find a store or restaurant when I need one."

Interestingly, many of these same people have, at some time in their lives, toted around special diet foods with great pride. Why is it okay to carry diet foods to the office but not the foods we really desire?

Compulsive eaters are embarrassed by their need to eat and their interest in food. Because they've spent their lives attempting to keep their eating a secret, they feel that carrying a food bag constitutes going public. "How can I take food with me when everyone around me thinks I should be dieting?" people ask us.

Remarkably, most compulsive eaters who reach this point in our program are readier than they know. They discover, for example, that among the people most interested in the food they carry are those whose reactions they most feared. One woman told us, "This afternoon I got hungry and reached into my desk drawer for some cashews. When I noticed the woman at a desk close to mine looking at me, I felt very uncomfortable. Then she said, 'I *love* cashews. May I have a few?' That was the end of that."

When you think about it without making judgments, the idea of carrying "something for the road" makes a great deal of sense. To pull it off, however, you have to remind yourself that your embarrassment stems from a feeling of nonentitlement and that, to the contrary, you are entitled. Eating is not a transgression. It is your basic right.

Some people are more resentful than embarrassed about carrying food around. "That's ridiculous," they say when the subject of a food bag comes up. "I can't go to the trouble of packing up my kitchen every time I leave the house." Their tone invariably suggests that packing a food bag is an enormous chore.

In truth, their resentment has more to do with having to care for themselves than with the specifics of packing a bag of food. They are reluctant to take on the job of reparenting themselves, perhaps equating parenting with resentment. Maybe their parents let them know that they weren't worth the trouble and they've assumed the same attitude about themselves. Either way, compulsive eaters who resent the prospect of carrying the foods they need have to come to terms with their resentment before they can resolve their addiction to food. If you are going to become your own authority about your eating, you have to take charge, and providing for yourself by carrying food is essential to the process.

Making Peace with the Food Bag: Experience indicates that our initial resistance to carrying food is short-lived. People who become accustomed to a food bag often say that they would no sooner leave home without it than without their wallet. "It's funny," one woman told us. "At first I felt self-conscious about packing my favorite foods in my purse, but now I'm so used to it that I can't imagine going out without it. Before, I'd get hungry, look around to see what I could find to eat, and settle for whatever was available, but I never felt satisfied when I compromised that way. Now I get hungry, I eat what I want, and I go on with my life. I wouldn't have it any other way. It's so natural that I can't imagine why I ever found the idea repugnant."

Again, the purpose of carrying food is to make sure that something you like is at hand when you're hungry. Sometimes you'll have exactly what you want; other times you'll have to compromise. If you don't have exactly what you want, we suggest you eat just a bite or two to quiet your hunger until you can get what you prefer.

The idea of carrying the food you like and eating it whenever you're hungry rather than sitting down to three square meals a day represents a whole new style of eating. It has been described by the media as "grazing," and we are pleased to report that grazing appears to be the wave of the future.

Humans, the Grazing Animals

As you begin to pay attention to stomach hunger and take the foods you like with you wherever you go, you will probably find yourself eating more often during the day. We are highly suspicious of those who report, at this phase of their development, that they just weren't hungry for anything other than breakfast, lunch, and dinner. We know that it's difficult to break with tradition and allow your stomach, not the clock, to guide you. We also recognize that human beings are natural grazers.

Given the opportunity, people who work long hours and have little time to shop, cook, and eat, tend to grab one bite here and another there. Our consumer society facilitates this new eating style by providing all sorts of fast-food eateries. Old-fashioned full-service restaurants have been joined by specialty stands serving baked potatoes, pizza, popcorn, and sushi. All these facilities are thriving as a result of this new way of eating. Instead of sitting down for steak and potatoes, today's eater may prefer to stand up for a potato with cheese, sour cream, or chives. Grazing—eating small amounts of food when you want them—has become chic, and it appears that demand feeding will be the wave of the future. At long last, you and your culture's eating style will be in sync.

There will be times, of course, when you'll want to eat dinner rather than graze, and you may even find that you like to eat a full dinner every night. If you make that discovery by genuinely attending to your hunger, it's perfectly fine. All we are urging is that you allow yourself the freedom to experiment and discover *when* you get hungry.

– 11 –

What to Eat

After you learn to identify the sensation of stomach hunger, you'll have to learn to identify exactly what kind of food best satisfies your need. To discover this you must ask "What am I hungry for?" Answering this question requires that you learn to make a match between your feeling of hunger and a particular food, to "read your hunger."

Reading your hunger involves, first, giving up the rules that govern food choices. We have accustomed ourselves to the notion that cereal, toast, eggs, and juice are "good" breakfast foods; that sandwiches, soup, and salads are for lunch; and that meat, fish, and a variety of vegetables make for a proper dinner. We have even specified the order in which food should be eaten within a given meal. For example, soup is always first and dessert last. A child of five can tell you that vegetables are "what you have to eat before you get dessert."

Conventions like these preclude the possibility of eating in response to natural desires. If, for example, you wake up one morning hungry for the turkey and stuffing you put away after last night's dinner but don't regard that as suitable breakfast food, you will probably prepare a bowl of corn-flakes instead of unwrapping your leftovers. Similarly, if you're an "appropriate" eater who is in the mood for oatmeal with brown sugar and cream at dinnertime, chances are you'll make yourself eat a plateful of turkey and vegetables. If, however, you make a commitment to eat what you want when you are hungry, your "inappropriate" desires become real options for you.

Interestingly, we have found that much overeating is caused by people's dogged adherence to eating traditions and consequent failure to read their hunger properly. Because of that, most compulsive eaters who attempt to deny their cravings by eating "what they should" usually end up eating what they originally wanted *in addition to* what they should.

Imagine that you are hungry for sweets at 6:00 P.M., but decide to eat dinner instead. You eat soup, fish, broccoli, and a salad. When you finish all that, you still don't feel satisfied, so you help yourself to seconds. By then you're feeling stuffed, but still not satisfied. Next, dessert is offered, and no matter how stuffed you feel, you dig in. When you've finished your dessert you finally feel stuffed *and* satisfied. Had you eaten only the dessert, you would have consumed much less, avoided the uncomfortable stuffed feeling, and, of course, satisfied your particular hunger.

With all due respect to the wisdom of our five-year-olds who have already internalized the mores of our culture vis-à-vis eating, you are not obligated to eat vegetables before you can have dessert. Unfortunately, the rules we and our children have learned about eating have more to do with denying specific hungers than with responding to them.

The Nutrition Question

The great fear about eating what you're hungry for is that you will suffer nutritionally. Traditional wisdom has it that we must be taught what to eat and eat what we're taught.

Such is not the case. We believe that your body knows best exactly what foods it needs at any given moment.

It is important to recognize that the body is really self-regulatory. Your body can tell you when to eat and exactly what food will meet your hunger need at any given moment. Numerous studies have concluded that self-directed young children have the capacity to eat healthfully.

Based on a series of experiments that have come to be called the "cafeteria studies," Dr. Clara Davis concluded that, left to their own devices, young babies choose all the foods they need to ensure healthy growth and development. Nutritional scientists are recommending that, instead of focusing on what we eat at any given meal, or even over the course of a day, we look at our diets over the span of a week or two and decide whether we are getting the nutrients necessary for good health.

These studies suggest that while you may choose to eat potatoes for lunch and dinner today, by tomorrow or the next day you will probably crave salads. At another time your body will crave meat or other foods that will balance your diet. If you eat what your body craves, rather than attempt to convince yourself that you should eat something else, you'll find that over a relatively short period of time you will vary your intake and eat what you need. You will meet all of your nutritional requirements if you trust your internal cues and respond specifically to them. Apparently, three meals a day chosen carefully from the basic food groups isn't worth the proverbial can of beans—if the can of beans is what you really want.

Matchmaking in Theory

You learn to identify what you're hungry for by asking yourself, "What food will satisfy the sensation in my stomach right now?" You will want, of course, to eat something that satisfies your desire for taste and texture, but the most important issue is whether what you eat will satisfy the hunger that originates in your stomach.

Compulsive eaters often think that our discussion of matching a particular food with stomach hunger sounds strange. Noncompulsive eaters, however, know exactly what we're talking about. When a noncompulsive eater says "I feel like eating a steak tonight," she is really saying that her body craves steak. If you have genuinely legalized all foods, and if you ask yourself what, specifically, you are hungry for every time you feel stomach hunger, you will be able to make a good match. You will picture the first food that comes to mind and try to see what it would feel like in your stomach. Is it the right weight and texture? Is it too hot or too cold? Too bland or too spicy? Your stomach knows that foods have different tastes, textures, and consistencies. It recognizes the difference between proteins, carbohydrates, fruits, and vegetables, but it doesn't make value judgments about each category. It simply knows what it wants, and when you satisfy it, your stomach will let you know that it's happy. This is how it works.

You're hungry. You think first about a roast beef sandwich and imagine that sandwich in your stomach. Does it feel right to you? If not, what's wrong with it? Is it too heavy? The idea of the sandwich may be appealing, but if it's not right for your stomach at that moment, you'll need to find an alternative. If roast beef feels too heavy when you think about it, try thinking of something lighter. Scrambled eggs? Getting close, but the eggs alone feel too light. Scrambled eggs on a roll? If you learn to try a variety of foods in your imagination each time you're hungry, you will eventually be able to zero in on exactly what you want. Should you not have that particular food with you, you'll be able to substitute something similar or have a few bites of something else until you get the food you want.

Some people find that their food cravings run in cycles—they crave one or two foods for a while, then suddenly feel a need for something different. It's not unusual, for example, for people to report that they seem to be on a "white food" cycle—cheese, pasta, chicken. Just as they begin to wonder if they'll ever want to eat a green vegetable again, the urge for one strikes, and they feed it.

An exciting article by Trish Hall in the *New York Times Magazine*, September 27, 1987, entitled "Cravings," reported that many studies are being done on the relationship between physiology and the foods we choose to eat. Although the data are inconclusive, both animal and human studies suggest that we crave the foods we need.

Is There Life After Chocolate?

"If I eat whatever I want when I'm hungry," Lila said before she embarked on a program of demand eating, "all I'll ever eat will be chocolate and ice cream. How can I *not* gain weight when I eat chocolate all the time?"

It's not hard to see why Lila, and compulsive eaters like her, imagine themselves living exclusively on chocolate—or some other formerly forbidden food—if they allow themselves to match what they eat with their specific hunger. Most compulsive eaters have spent their lives craving foods they were not allowed, foods that are usually high in calories. When they think about eating what they want, their minds automatically flash to those forbidden goodies. In the beginning, most of you will probably eat large amounts of those foods that were formerly forbidden.

Lila, from her ongoing reports, was no exception. "I waited to get hungry and each time my hunger hit," she told us, "I wanted a chocolate milk shake. I would drive to my favorite coffee shop, order two of them, and go. On the one hand, I felt like a milk shake addict; on the other, I felt great. At one period I was drinking an average of two milk shakes a day. I'd wait until I was hungry, which was usually around eleven-thirty A.M., and I'd have my milk shakes. At some point I started to worry about my weight, but when I thought about my eating I had an interesting realization. Before I started this approach I'd have had my routine breakfast at eight A.M. and a sandwich and diet Coke at lunchtime. Now I don't eat that breakfast or that lunch and just have my milk shakes. I'm actually eating less than I used to and enjoying it more."

After a month of milk shakes, Lila's cravings began to change. Although it seemed to her at the onset that her interest in milk shakes would never fade, once she convinced herself that she could have one whenever she was hungry for it, Lila's desires for other foods surfaced.

When you begin to work at matchmaking you have to open yourself to experimentation. You may find yourself eating all kinds of foods that defy convention. You may even find yourself eating foods you've always considered unhealthy. If you're worried about your health, take a daily vitamin to reassure yourself. We think you'll be surprised to find, however, that your desire for vegetables is hiding just beneath the milk shakes. Indeed, the surprise for people who have allowed themselves to be ruled by diets is that when they make an accurate match, their bodies return to their natural, usually lower weight.

A Weighty Issue

Whenever we talk about eating whatever you want at the moment you are hungry, we find ourselves face to face with the issue of weight. "What's going to happen to my weight?"

is a question that lurks in the minds of all compulsive eaters all of the time.

As demand feeding replaces your compulsive eating you will see changes in your weight. Remember that when you tune in to your body, you are turning over to it the process of weight loss, allowing your body to tell you when, what, and how much to eat. Once you do this, you will begin to return to what, for you, is a natural weight. In other words, once you've broken your addiction to food, once food on demand replaces compulsive eating, your body will reflect the change.

Compulsive eaters fall into two general categories with regard to weight. They are either much heavier than their natural weight as a result of the diet/binge cycle or much lighter than their natural weight as a result of ongoing deprivation. If you've managed to maintain an artificially low weight through diets, you may gain some weight once you lift all food bans. It's crucial, however, not to think of that weight gain as the sort that comes from binging. You will stop gaining weight when your body reaches its setpoint—the weight you were "designed" to have. If you find yourself gaining a great deal of weight it is probably because you are secretly threatening to withhold food from yourself and therefore stoking up for the upcoming deprivation.

If you weigh much more than your natural weight you will begin to lose weight when you eat from stomach hunger. Your excess weight is the result of eating when you aren't hungry or eating foods you aren't hungry for or eating more food than your stomach wants. When you stop that kind of eating, your weight will drop, provided that your metabolism has not been too damaged by dieting. Your weight will eventually settle in at an amount that conforms to your genetic program.

Some of you will discover that the years of dieting have taken a toll on your metabolism and that you would have to eat considerably less than your body needs in order to lose weight. People who discover how harmful dieting has been are justifiably angry. Hopefully, if your weight does not change significantly, you will still experience great relief in breaking your addiction to food.

What happens with your weight will depend a great deal on the extent to which you've renounced the diet/binge cycle. If you are scrupulous about eating what you want when you are hungry, if you know that regardless of the outcome you will never again diet or yell at yourself for your eating or your weight, you have nothing to fear. The evidence is overwhelming: *The more relaxed you are about your need to eat, the less you will eat.*

Matchmaking in Action

Ruth told us that she had finally begun to get the hang of reading her hunger. "Yesterday afternoon I was hungry," she explained, "and thought that I wanted something sweet. I'm a chocoholic, and the first thing that came to mind was chocolate. I thought about a chocolate brownie, but when I imagined eating it, I realized that it was too sweet, too heavy, and too chewy. I thought about cookies and then about cake, but neither seemed quite right. Then I remembered how much I used to love pudding when I was a kid. I hadn't had any in years. As soon as I thought about it, I remembered that the deli near my office had a sign advertising homemade rice pudding. I was sure it would be the perfect match—it's sweet and light and just the right texture and I have all sorts of good memories about it. I think that rice pudding is going to be a staple of my diet for a while."

Arthur had a similarly successful, although different experience. "It was Saturday morning," he told us, "and I woke up feeling very hungry. My first thought was that I wanted something really substantial, like pancakes and bacon. But when I tried to imagine eating the pancakes I realized that they weren't really what I wanted. I imagined them in my stomach and just didn't feel satisfied. I did the same thing with the bacon and had a negative reaction. The salt and the grease were just wrong. At that point I began to think about different sorts of food. I considered oatmeal and omelettes, but they weren't right. Finally, I realized that what I wanted was something good and chewy. I tried out a bagel and it was perfect. But I needed something with it, some protein. Cream cheese didn't do it, but it was close. After imagining a few other things I finally came to the idea of a toasted bagel with melted cheese. It seemed just perfect, so I made it and ate it, and sure enough, it *was* perfect!"

Arthur added that in the past he would have eaten the pancakes and bacon that had first occurred to him. He would have stuffed himself in an effort to feel satisfied. "But I realize now," he explained, "that no matter how much I eat of something I don't want, I won't find it satisfying. Before I began matching my hunger with specific foods, I overate all the time. After stuffing myself with pancakes and bacon I would have spent the rest of the day eating whatever I came across, just because I wasn't satisfied. Now that I think about what I want and eat it, I feel more satisfied with much less food."

Some Complications

It isn't always easy to learn to match your hunger with a specific food. Many people have a hard time, especially at the beginning. Often it's just a matter of trial and error until you get the hang of it. Sometimes, however, the problem is a bit more complicated.

Andrea found it nearly impossible to rid herself of the calorie chart that years of dieting had etched into her brain. "You name a food," she told us, "and the first thing that pops into my mind is a number. I don't feel that I can really make a free choice about what I want with all those numbers getting in the way."

Others have trouble freeing themselves of traditional notions about meals. "The idea of just eating dessert, even if it's what I really crave," said one man, "is something I couldn't possibly do. Even if I'm hungry for ice cream when I wake up in the morning, it just wouldn't feel right to me to eat it."

When you can't find anything that makes the match—and there will be such times—we suggest that you check to be sure you're really hungry. If you are, eat a small amount of something bland or nondescript. Don't expect bells to ring with each eating experience. Keep in mind that you are trying to eat out of stomach hunger as many times a day as possible. When you can't make the perfect match at any given moment, don't eat a great deal of something less than perfect, and you'll have another opportunity to match your hunger with a particular food before long. However, if you discover that you really aren't hungry, we suggest that you not eat anything. Just wait fifteen minutes and take another reading.

Once you've learned to read your hunger, your matching technique will become fairly automatic. You'll discover the certain pleasure that comes from making the perfect match between your hunger and what you eat. Eating is one of the few areas in life in which you can get exactly what you wish for most of the time. If you want the crust on the rye bread, we urge you to forget about the inside part. If you want dessert, skip the meat and potatoes. If you're longing for the thick chocolate frosting on a piece of devil's food cake, eat the frosting and leave the cake. And make certain to be specific when you choose a brand. We all know that no two brands of chocolate chip cookies taste the same.

As you try to figure out what you want to eat, it helps to provide yourself with as great a variety of choices as possible. There will be times, of course, when you just don't have what you want, and at those times you'll have to come as close to your wish as you can. If you're hungry for clams at midnight and you don't have any, you don't have to go clamming. Think about the taste and texture of clams— about how they'd feel in your stomach—and try to come up with an alternative. Hamburger, obviously, won't do as well as tuna fish.

Another problem that arises when you try to match your hunger with a particular food is very practical: How do you plan meals ahead of time if your hunger is tied to a particular moment? You can't possibly know at 7:00 A.M. what you'll want to eat at 7:00 P.M. Needless to say, the more food you have from which to choose, the easier it is to organize meals that are tied to your hunger. As you become a more proficient matchmaker, however, you'll develop a better sense of which foods you most frequently crave. They will become your staples, and you'll make a point of having them around in ample quantity.

We will deal with making choices when you're eating out in a later chapter. For the moment it is enough to remember that when you eat in a restaurant you should consult your stomach *before* you consult a menu.

Remember

When you begin to read your hunger, don't expect to choose food that resembles a "traditional" meal. When you ask your stomach what it's hungry for, it doesn't usually respond with a choice of appetizer, entrée, vegetable, and dessert. It's considerably less sophisticated than that. Your stomach will usually give you one strong signal. Listen carefully and try to respond to it as specifically as you can. Matching your hunger with a particular food won't give you the meal of a lifetime, but it affords you all sorts of exciting eating experiences.

How Much to Eat

How Much Is Enough?

Learning when you've had enough to eat is just a variation of learning when you're hungry. It requires tuning into the signals your stomach sends you. If, as you eat, your stomach becomes full, it will stop sending hunger signals, and you can stop eating. If, as you eat, your stomach continues to send hunger signals, it means that you haven't had enough.

The idea of hunger signals may sound a bit strange to you, but once you begin to experience them they will probably feel familiar. Do infants turn away from the bottle or breast when they've had enough? Sometimes they finish the bottle, sometimes they leave it half full, and sometimes they finish it, cry for more, and get it tout de suite. In every case, their appetite, rather than the size of the bottle, determines how much they drink. Unfortunately, as most infants make the transition to solid foods, their right to decide how much is enough is no longer respected. Adults become increasingly concerned about what and how much children eat. "One spoonful for Grandma" and the Clean Plate Club are signs of the ubiquitous household battle for the title Boss of Eating.

Most of you, for example, have a membership in the Clean Plate Club dating back to childhood. The only membership requirement was that you finish everything you were served. Lest you not take this requirement seriously, an appeal may have been made to your conscience. "There are children starving in Africa/Armenia/Europe/Ethiopia." Somehow, by eating everything placed before you, you were doing your part to help those children or showing proper appreciation for being spared their suffering. The issue of your sense of fullness clearly took a back seat to the issues of clean plates and global starvation.

It's hard to resist poking fun at these feeding techniques, but we must recognize that our mothers, and their mothers before them, had our best interests at heart. It was their job to prepare meals to nurture us, and they were rewarded when we ate. However, as you attempt to reestablish the connection between hunger and eating, it's important for you to look at the impact the Clean Plate Club and the evocation of starving children had on your eating behavior.

"Whenever I left anything on my plate," recalled June, forty-five, "my mother would look me in the eye and tell me that there were little girls in Europe who were starving and that I should finish every bite. I remember at some point trying to make a connection. I must have been five when I asked in all seriousness if we could send my leftover hamburger to them. My mother laughed and said that it couldn't be done. I don't know exactly what happened then, but I know that whenever I pushed away a plate with anything on it, I felt bad."

Although on one level June was puzzled, on another she understood that she was dealing with frustration—her mother's at having prepared something that went uneaten—and the threat implied in "remember the starving" that if June wasn't grateful and didn't express her gratitude by eating everything on her plate, she might be numbered among the starving. Although June's mother never intended to threaten her, mother and daughter were enmeshed in a socially sanctioned battle for control over who would determine how much was enough.

Becoming the Boss of Your Own Eating

Before you can become the boss of your own eating, before you can learn to determine for yourself when you've had enough, you must develop an acute awareness of all the ways in which you currently relinquish that authority.

What Constitutes a Serving: You go out for dinner and order an entrée of prime ribs, baked potato, garden fresh carrots, and an endive salad. When the food arrives you see before you two large, thick slices of beef, one on a bone, a big baked potato split down the middle and filled with sour cream, about half a cup of carrots, and a wooden bowl, about eight inches in diameter, filled with greens. You're hungry and you dig in. After about twenty minutes you begin to feel full, but you look at your plate and see that you've barely touched the potato, half the carrots are still there, and you have a way to go on the meat. The salad bowl, however, is empty. What do you do?

Most compulsive eaters take a deep breath and continue to eat. After all, their logic goes, they haven't finished their "serving." The time has come to question how a serving is determined. Can it be that whoever put the food on your plate knows how much you need to eat better than you yourself do? Suppose you finish the food on your plate and want more? The implication is that there is something right about the quantities you were served, and something wrong about the quantities you want.

Your concern about servings suggests that the potter who

designed your dinnerware had some special knowledge of how much you'd need to eat when you sat down for dinner and the baker knew how much bread you'd want when he shaped his rolls. But what the restaurateur deems to be a serving may or may not be the amount of food you require at a particular moment. Serving sizes have nothing to do with you and satiety.

When you're eating with other people, you'll notice that noncompulsive eaters often leave some food on their plates. At some point in the future you will be among them, and you'll do it without even thinking about it. To get to that point, however, you must reclaim the title of boss and make your own how-much decisions from the inside out.

Technique: The following techniques are all designed to help you learn to listen to your stomach for "full" signals.

- *Take a few bites, then stop eating.* Are you still hungry? If you are, take a few more bites and stop again. Are you satisfied yet? Sometimes it's helpful to take a break and walk around for a while before you come back to the question of hunger. When you can finally answer yes, to the question of whether you've had enough, the time has come to stop eating.
- *Experiment with your sensation of fullness.* There are varying levels of satiety. You can eat until you no longer feel the hunger signal at all, you can eat until you feel a certain level of satisfaction, or you can eat until you feel full.You can also eat beyond fullness to feeling stuffed. Each of us has a different point at which we are ready to stop eating. You'll need to find the one that feels most comfortable for you and be certain that you don't make all sorts of judgments about what that point is. Some people, for example, have to feel stuffed to feel safe—food, and fullness in

particular, represent much more than simple physical satiation. We refer to the need to feel very full as a need for psychological rather than physiological fullness. Just as you had to move from mouth hunger to stomach hunger, you will have to move in the direction of physical fullness if you expect to rediscover your natural weight. As with mouth hunger, however, you cannot simply will yourself to stop eating as soon as you are physiologically full. The shift will not occur until you have established an accepting, caring environment in which you can learn how much is enough for you.

It's So Hard to Say Good-bye

Many of us have difficulty with partings. As a compulsive eater, you may discover that your difficulty with good-byes extends to food. Those who have an addictive relationship to food endow it with all kinds of meaning. Food may be a friend or a trusted companion that makes you feel safe, in which case you will probably be as reluctant to part with it as you would be to part with someone near and dear.

Once you have legalized foods, however, concern over saying good-bye is greatly diminished. As soon as you recognize that all foods are legal and accessible, that you can have as much of any one food as you want, you'll also understand that good-bye is not forever. You have the luxury of deciding how much you want at any given moment because you have pledged to give yourself more when you need it.

Alice was a guest at a wedding shower. She loved the entrée, fish stuffed with shrimp and crabmeat and topped with an extraordinary sauce. The hostess served generous portions and Alice was enjoying it thoroughly. About halfway through, she realized that she was no longer hungry. "In the past," Alice explained, "I would have continued eating. I couldn't possibly have stopped before my plate was empty. This time, however, I did two things. Telling the hostess that I thought it was delicious, I asked if I might take the rest home with me and asked her for the recipe before I left. I realized that I could make it for myself anytime, and didn't have to eat any more than I wanted."

Alice benefited in two ways from being in touch with her stomach. First, she developed an awareness of how much fish she was hungry for in one sitting. And second, she was able to really enjoy the fish that she ate. Consuming more than you are hungry for interferes with the pleasure of eating.

Interestingly, the primary reason to stop eating when you've had enough is to be able to return to food soon. Remember that as you learn to eat from stomach hunger, your goal is to accumulate checks on the stomach hunger side of your ledger, which means that you must try to feed yourself on demand as often as possible. If you say good-bye to food at just the right moment, you'll be in a good position to say hello to it again before long.

Alice's impulse to ask to take the fish home was a good one. Much overeating results from the fear that if you don't eat everything right away, it won't be there later when you want it. If you take it with you, you can be sure that it *will* be there. It's not unusual to discover that if you stop eating as soon as you're full, your hunger returns very quickly. If it does, you'll have to figure out what you're hungry for. If it's what you were eating, and you have access to it, you can satisfy your hunger easily.

Some people cultivate the habit of leaving at least a mouthful of whatever they're eating on the plate. When you're trying to learn about fullness, this can help to remind you to focus on finding a pleasurable way to say good-bye.

Feeling Satisfied with Less

When people learn to stop eating when they're full, they often discover that their bodies need much less food than they thought. "I notice that after a few bites I really could stop," they say. "I've had enough but I push on. I just don't want to stop after I've had so little."

Some people feel reluctant to stop eating when they notice they've had enough because they're discomfited by the realization that so little food could satisfy their hunger. Having always thought they needed "a lot," they are disoriented by feeling satisfied with "a little."

Other people panic when they realize how little they'd be eating if they stopped each time they felt full. "Can I really sustain myself with so little food?" they ask. The answer, of course, is that the body is self-regulatory and they've been overeating for a long time. If they can ride out their fear, they will become more comfortable with eating less.

Another group of compulsive eaters object on still different grounds to stopping when they've had enough. "I don't like the idea that I'm going to spend the rest of my life eating so little. Food, after all, is very pleasurable and I want to enjoy it." What this group cannot know at the beginning of this process is that one's food requirements change over time. If you've been overeating, you require much less food to reach your natural weight. Your weight will eventually stabilize, your food needs will change accordingly, and you will eat more.

Sweet Farewells

When you're really tuned in to fullness, you'll notice that at times you feel full but still want something sweet to finish off the eating experience. The urge for something sweet, even after a satisfying meal, is a common one. That's why most cultures provide desserts. If you are really living free in a world of food, it shouldn't present a problem.

The urge for a sweet dessert usually has nothing to do with stomach hunger. In fact, some people discover that when they legalize foods, their stomach hunger rarely turns them toward sweets. One woman said, "Every time I'm hungry I really attempt to imagine how different foods will feel in my stomach. Chocolate ice cream, which was my nemesis for years, seems too sweet most of the time. Here I've gone and made ice cream equal to lettuce in my mind, and I'm never really all that hungry for ice cream. It seems unfair that now that I'm allowing myself the thing I've always craved, I'm never hungry for it."

If, for you, sweets are seldom a match for stomach hunger, dessert is a place where they may fit in with your new way of eating. Since the urge to eat something sweet after a meal has nothing to do with stomach hunger, you have to approach your urge for sweets differently than most other eating and think more in terms of your mouth. This time when you ask "What would I like to eat?" you're trying to decide what taste in what form you'd like to experience: ice, ice cream, candy, pie, cake, mousse, fruit, liqueur?

As you become more experienced at allowing yourself a sweet farewell, you'll probably discover that it takes only a bite or two to satisfy your urge. Remember, if you aren't eating to fill your stomach, you probably won't have to eat much. When sweets are no longer forbidden, you'll find nothing extraordinary about having a few bites. You're only after the taste of sweetness, and you can always come back for more if you want it. Of course, if you decide in advance that you want more than a small sampling of dessert, you'll plan to save room for a larger portion. As always, you're the boss.

Fine-Tuning When, What, and How Much

People generally master the problems of when, what, and how much to eat in that order. It takes a while to become an attuned feeder. Although you may be tempted to say "Great! Now I have the answer. I'm going to eat only when I'm hungry, exactly what I want, in the amounts I want," it would be impossible for you to simply start feeding yourself accurately without a hitch. That would be akin to putting yourself on a diet. You would be attempting to control, rather than cure, your compulsive need for food.

Remember that you are nudging yourself in the direction of stomach hunger. As you become more able to address the questions accurately, you will see a decrease in your need to eat from mouth hunger. As a result, most of you will begin to return to your natural weight. During the transition from compulsive eating to finely tuned demand feeding, certain situations may be a bit difficult. Chapter 13 will walk you through them.

– 13 –

Everyday Life as a Demand Feeder

Although demand feeding is the most natural, reasonable way for human beings to eat, much of our day-to-day life is structured in a way that, at first glance at least, appears to complicate the process. These complications are best resolved if we look at them in terms of the questions compulsive eaters have asked us over the years.

Q. I've spent most of my life on diets, always feeling out of step with the rest of the world regarding eating. My friends would be eating a burger and fries while I was eating grapefruit. It seems as if demand feeding is just one more way for me to be out of step. Will the time ever come when I can really eat normally?

A. We define "normal" as eating when you're hungry, what you're hungry for, and stopping when you've had enough. Most noncompulsive eaters are able to divide their eating experiences into breakfast, lunch, and dinner because they've trained themselves to get hungry at those prescribed hours. If you listen to noncompulsive eaters for a while, however, you'll hear the catch phrases of demand feeding.

- Thanks, but I'm not hungry right now.
- I've eaten, but I'll be happy to sit with you while you eat something.
- Gee, it was delicious and I'd love more, but I'm really too full.
- It looks wonderful, but I think I'll wait for my entrée. If I eat that now, I won't be hungry when my order arrives.
- I'm full. I'm going to ask the waiter to pack up the rest so I can take it home.

Noncompulsive eaters manage to conform to social norms without straying from their hunger signals. To be sure, they may occasionally eat until they feel stuffed or pop something into their mouths "just because it looks good," but when they do, they don't regard it as a big deal. They complain about how full they are and then forget about it. Food, for them, may range in importance from necessary to pleasurable to exquisite, but it is not something magical and forbidden that must be kept off limits or swallowed whole.

There will come a time when you will be able to arrange your hunger to better coincide with traditional mealtimes if you want to. However, it's important to stay as free of "outside" eating schedules as you possibly can, when you begin to search for your identity as an eater. It's hard enough to figure out when you're hungry and what you're hungry for without having the added burden of conforming to someone else's schedule and desires. During this period of discovery, which puts you on the road toward "normal" eating, you'll have to determine for yourself whether you're more comfortable eating alone or in the company of others at a so-called meal. The key is to stay aware of and attuned to your hunger.

Q. If I only eat when I'm hungry, what happens to the pleasure of going to a restaurant? Your approach is supposed to avoid deprivation, but I'd feel deprived if I had to give up going out to eat with my friends.

A. Eating what you want when you're hungry is easiest when you're at home or in the privacy of your office. Moving your new mode of eating into the public arena of a restaurant does raise all sorts of issues. Fortunately, they can all be resolved quite easily. We'll begin with an assurance that, indeed, you can go out to eat in a restaurant with friends even if you are learning to feed yourself on demand. Let's look at what dining out means in terms of when, what, and how much.

When you agree to meet someone for a meal in a restaurant, you're forgoing the choice of when to eat and opting instead for companionship and the easy pleasure of a meal out. The potential conflict of making dates to eat out is that you want to be hungry for your meal, but you don't want to ignore any hunger signals you might feel earlier. If you have a one o'clock lunch date, for example, but feel hungry at noon, you have to figure out a way to respond to your early hunger and still be hungry when you get to the restaurant.

You want to have it both ways and you can. At noon, you simply say "I'm hungry now. What can I eat to address my hunger that will allow me to be hungry again when I get to the restaurant?" If, for example, you are into bread and cheese, you might take a few bites of a buttered roll with cheese. After you've eaten a small amount, you can wait a few minutes and check in with your hunger again. With practice, you will learn just how much food it takes to satisfy your hunger of the moment without closing the door on hunger an hour hence.

There is always the possibility that you will arrive at a restaurant for a meal and not be hungry. If you haven't been able to "arrange" your hunger to accommodate your schedule, you will have to learn how to say "I thought I'd be hungry by this time, but I'm not. Please go ahead and order. I'll just have something to drink, and if I get hungry later, I'll order then." If the restaurant has a minimum charge for each person, you can pay it or order something to take home.

A restaurant is an ideal place to ask yourself "*What* do I want to eat?" The options are usually greater when you go out than they are at home. The key, again, is to check in with your stomach *before* you open the menu.

The problem new demand feeders encounter most frequently in a restaurant has more to do with external expectations than with hunger. Somehow, expectations as to what one should eat and the order in which it should be eaten are heightened in a restaurant. If you consult your stomach before opening the menu you're less likely to be trapped by printed headings like APPETIZER, ENTRÉE, and DESSERT. You'll know before you begin to read if you're hungry for something sweet, something light, something major, and you can regard the menu as a smorgasbord from which to select. If you want a shrimp cocktail, a cup of coffee, and a piece of apple pie, order them. If your friends are having a light lunch but you want a steak, order that.

In an ideal world, your individual eating preferences would not constitute a problem. In the less than perfect world in which we live, however, someone may give you a hard time when you order what you really want. One woman told us that when she ordered an appetizer rather than a main course, she thought her waiter looked displeased. "I felt uncomfortable," she explained. "Then it occurred to me that his tips were usually calculated on the basis of the bill and that it took as much of his effort and time to wait on me as on someone who was ordering a full meal.

I figured that rather than feel uncomfortable, I'd address the problem straight on. So when he came back I explained that although I wasn't hungry, I fully intended to tip him on the basis of my stay, not my order. He showed embarrassment for a minute, but that quickly faded and he became extremely pleasant. We were both happy."

The answer to *how much* is the same in a restaurant as at home. Always eat as much as you are hungry for—not more, not less. Economics and custom, not the appetites of individual patrons, determine the sizes of restaurant portions. If, as you eat your meal, you check in with your hunger and discover that you want more, you can always ask to see the menu again. If, however, you discover that you aren't hungry enough to finish your entire serving, you should be prepared to leave what remains or ask to take it with you. It's not unusual, food prices being what they are, for people to take leftovers home for themselves, not the dog.

The key to all these situations is your feeling of entitlement. If you respect your needs, there's no reason why they should interfere with the needs of anyone else.

Q. It's one thing to sit out a meal in a restaurant, but what about when a friend invites you to her home for dinner? How do you deal with that?

A. If you believe that feeding yourself what you're hungry for when you want it is natural and necessary, you won't have trouble handling any social situation.

When you accept an invitation to dine at a friend's home, you're agreeing to be hungry at a predetermined time and to eat what your host prepares. You are saying that you will arrange to time your hunger for the pleasure of the evening, which is not difficult. We have already discussed techniques for ensuring that you will be hungry at a given time. Eating at someone's house differs from eating in a restaurant, however, because you have fewer options regarding what you eat.

What do you do? First, look at everything that is being served and determine what best suits your hunger of the moment. Assume, for example, that there's a big salad, beef Stroganoff, string beans, and rice and you've learned that frozen orange cognac soufflé is in the wings. The dessert is just what you want—cold, light, and not too sweet. The meat just doesn't do it for you—it's too heavy. The salad and rice are appealing. The string beans aren't right at all.

You really want to sustain your hunger until dessert, so you take just enough rice and salad to leave room and skip the meat and string beans. If you find it hard to pass on food because you're concerned about the host's response, help yourself to a small portion, which you can then taste or simply move around on your plate. If you're offered seconds, a simple "No thanks, I'm full" or "I'm saving room for dessert" usually suffices. You're probably not off base if you suspect that some hosts and hostesses want their dinner guests to show approval by taking more. If you feel pushed, you can always say "I really would love more, but I'm too full right now. If there's any left I'd be delighted to take some home and have it tomorrow." Asking for a recipe is also a nice way to say "I've had enough now, but I've enjoyed it."

Q. How do I stick to food on demand when I'm at a big, catered party?

A. People are often confused about what to do at big social gatherings where so much of the food looks inviting. We've discovered that the trouble usually stems from their having forgotten that no food is off limits. In other words, when surrounded by dozens of floating hors d'oeuvres trays filled with special goodies, a newcomer to demand feeding is apt to forget that one can have as much or as little of anything as one wants.

In these situations, it's important to remember that it's never pleasurable to eat something just because it's there, particularly when you're not hungry. If you find yourself faced with fabulous, tempting food, but your stomach is not hungry—and if, as with hors d'oeuvres at a wedding, you cannot realistically expect to take some home with you—you have to tell yourself "I hope that sometime when I'm hungry I'll be around such foods again" or "I must remember to think about getting some of these incredible-looking things when I'm hungry."

Let us tell you a story about a particularly gutsy way of handling the "special event." Nan wasn't the least bit hungry when the food was served at her cousin's wedding. The dinner was being held at a four-star restaurant. Nan knew the reputation of the place—and that she could not afford to eat there on her own—so she prepared herself to be hungry. The evening began with hors d'oeuvres, however, and Nan, who had been into light snack foods, flipped over them. She'd never had any that were so elaborate and good. By the time she sat down to the main meal, she realized that she was ready for dessert and didn't want the main course at all. She quietly asked the waiter, as he was clearing the table, if he would wrap up her meal. He looked surprised but didn't say anything. She noticed someone across the table looking at her oddly.

At the end of the evening the bride came over to Nan and said, "I heard that you had your meal wrapped up to go. Good for you. We paid a fortune for this affair. I'm so glad you'll get to enjoy it at home. I hate seeing all this food go to waste."

Q. How do I go about feeding myself on demand when I have a family to feed as well?

A. When you are eating on demand and the rest of your family is eating as they always have, the problems are twofold. First, you won't know in advance what you want to eat, and, assuming that you are the one who prepares meals, chances are that you won't want to eat what you're making for everyone else. Second, it's unlikely that your hunger will always coincide with your family's eating schedule.

To keep yourself on course, you'll have to keep talking to yourself about your own hunger. That means continuing to reassure yourself that when you *are* hungry you will be able to have anything you want—the foods you've prepared for your family or anything else.

We recognize how difficult it is, at first, to sit with your family at mealtime and not eat, but it becomes easier. After a while everyone comes to recognize that you can share mealtimes without sharing meals. You can keep your family company while they're eating without partaking of anything yourself. Indeed, your own eating experience will be considerably more pleasant if you save it for a time when you are hungry.

Sue, the single parent of eleven-year-old twin daughters, told us:

"As a single mother I always placed enormous importance on dinnertime. I wanted it to be a wonderful time of sharing—sitting at the table, talking about our day, passing around a bowl of vegetables. Of course, it was never anything like that. I've always worked full time, then rushed home and tried to put together a respectable meal. The girls

*would be vying for my attention, and I'd feel irritated be-
cause my chicken wasn't done and my spinach had sand in
it and my potatoes were burning. Then we'd get to the table
and one of them would say that she wasn't hungry. The
other would say that the chicken didn't taste good. The apple
juice would spill. Someone might start to cry. All in all, the
calm, sharing times were few and far between.*

*"Still, the thought of not eating with them sent me into a
panic. It was hard to give up the fantasy of my respectable
family meal. What I discovered, once I stopped eating with
them, was that 'dinnertime' was a terrible time for me to
eat. I was too tense at the end of my workday to start putting
food into my stomach. I needed some time to unwind. Now
I simply prepare what they say they want, which is never
anything too elaborate—sometimes pizza, sometimes a hamburger. I can sit with them, relax, and enjoy them. Even
better, though, I get to enjoy my own dinner sitting alone
with a newspaper while they're off doing their homework. I
really didn't have to give up anything."*

Kids are one thing, but the issue of eating with a spouse is
another. "My husband tells me that he hates to eat alone,"
said Marilyn. "It's just not his idea of a good time." Marilyn
has several options. There will come a time when she'll be
able to work with her hunger so that she can have planned
'meals' with her husband. It will be hard for her to do this,
however, before she's had enough experience with stomach
hunger. Until then, she might try sitting with her husband
while he eats, ask him to postpone eating until she's hungry,
or find ways to spend time with him without sharing meals.
However she arranges it, she'll have to keep enough choices
of food on hand so they can each have what they're hungry
for when they eat.

Q. How do I go about turning my whole family on to demand feeding?

A. Before you begin to feed your entire family on demand—before you begin to share what you've learned about eating with them—you have to give yourself time to absorb all that you've learned about demand feeding. It's one thing to understand the idea of demand feeding intellectually and quite another to live with it. To make that leap you'll need time to experiment, to discover your own internal time clock, your own desires for food, and your own capacity. You won't be able to determine any of these things for yourself if you're focused on converting your family.

The time will come, to be sure, when you will be in a position to restructure your family's eating, if that's what you all want to do. When it does, you'll want to figure out how best it can work in your family. *Are You Hungry?* by Jane R. Hirschmann and Lela Zaphiropoulos can help.

One workshop participant told us how she handled the situation. "After I had been on this approach for a few months, I decided that it would be a good idea if my whole family—my husband and three children—were to eat on demand. One thing that I know will never change is that I do all the cooking and shopping. But I've decided that from now on I'll cook one hot meal a day for whoever wants it. I put dinner, from soup to nuts, on the table, and people can choose from what's there if they're hungry. If they don't want to eat, that's fine with me; if they want something else, they can get it themselves. It's all so relaxed and I'm thrilled to no longer be a nutritional drill sergeant."

Martha told us her story. "My changeover to demand feeding coincided with redoing my kitchen. I decided to break through to our dining room to make a family room where we could all cook, eat, and relax together. I also decided to cook foods that are easily reheated and have plenty of finger foods, as well as dessert items, available and to serve the food smorgasbord style. We can always find something we like because of the wide variety available. Our new-style family room is enjoyed by all."

Josephine, the mother of one teenage boy, said, "I told Jonathan that I was embarking on a new program to gain control of my eating and that I would need to have my own supply of food, which he shouldn't eat. Of course I felt guilty telling him this, so I decided to put a shopping list on the fridge and told him to add to it the special foods he'd like me to buy for him. I brought in three gallons of my favorite ice creams and one gallon of his. Yesterday he said, 'Ma, I don't know what kind of diet you're on now, but let me tell you this is by far the best one. I hope you don't go off it!' "

Q. Can I continue a demand-feeding schedule while I'm pregnant? After all, my physician/midwife has given me a list of the foods I need to eat daily to ensure the health of my baby. Doesn't this conflict with your approach?

A. What you are really asking is "Can I trust myself to eat properly while I'm pregnant?" The answer is a resounding yes! Why should your body fail you now? It's quite the reverse. Your body is going to tell you exactly what you need for both you and the baby. It's your job to listen carefully and follow the signals you receive.

Many pregnant women report that "the food charts handed to me at my first obstetric appointment made me crazy. If I tried to eat everything recommended, I'd be eating all day long." We suggest that, barring any medical contraindications, you work toward allowing your body to direct your eating during this nine-month period. You can always compare what you are eating naturally with the recommended diet. We think that if you follow your natural inclinations, over time you'll eat what you most need. If there are great discrepancies between what you want and what you think you should have, by all means talk it over with your physician.

Your eating will, of course, change from what has been your normal pattern. You will go through periods when you are eating larger quantities, your food selections may vary, and you may eat more frequently than usual. You may not crave pickles and ice cream, but you will find that you have particular cravings in response to your body's varying requirements. Remember that all these changes serve a purpose. Be aware of the shifts and respond accordingly.

Of course, the big concern for most pregnant women, even if they've never been compulsive eaters, is weight gain during pregnancy. Unfortunately, you are weighed in at each doctor's visit, and the numbers on the scale take on a life of their own. It is difficult not to judge yourself in the old way for gaining weight, but you must try.

Pregnancy weight has a purpose. Your body is housing a rapidly growing baby and preparing for the work of childbirth. The fat deposits on your hips and breasts are essential. Trust your body to tell you when, what, and how much you need to eat for a healthy pregnancy. And don't be surprised if you don't immediately bounce back to your prepregnancy weight. Whether you do or don't has a lot to do with your age and physical makeup. Just remember that your body won't fail you if you tune in to your internal signals of hunger and satiety.

Q. You are proposing that if I eat only when, what, and how much my body dictates, I'll return to what, for me, is a natural weight. Yet everyone these days suggests that exercise is crucial to weight loss. Do I need to embark on an exercise program along with demand feeding?

A. Remember that demand feeding is an antidote for compulsive eating. The weight loss that follows breaking your addiction to food is really a by-product of your work on this major problem. Depending on your particular body, exercise may enhance the possibility of weight loss, but it must always be approached with caution.

We are certainly in favor of exercising to feel better and look as good as one can. We are painfully aware, however, of how skillfully compulsive eaters weave exercise into their obsessions about eating and weight. When exercise is used to counteract calories it becomes yet another instrument of self-contempt and punishment. Exercise for the purpose of "getting rid of" parts of ourselves is bound to foment the same kind of rebellion that ends most diets. The graveyard of abandoned diets is strewn with unused health club memberships, exercise bicycles, and running shoes.

In order to exercise successfully, you will have to find a way to address these problems. First, your inspiration must flow from something other than "Yuck, I can't stand myself." Second, your exercise program must conform to you, not to some notion of who you think you should be. Like your eating, it must reflect your needs and preferences. If you impose a schedule and form of exercise on yourself that contains a hidden indictment of the current you, you will rebel.

Q. I have special problems—diabetes, high blood pressure, allergies—and as a result, I cannot eat certain foods without putting myself in jeopardy. I really can't live freely in a world of food. What should I do?

A. Many people have medical conditions that prohibit or limit their consumption of certain foods. Thay can feed themselves on demand, but they must limit themselves to foods their bodies can process properly.

Two factors are critical for such people. First, they must recognize that although their choice of foods may be limited, they can still use stomach hunger as a basis for eating. Even when they must key their eating to medication schedules, they can work toward some harmonious relationship with their natural hunger schedule.

Second, it is important for people with medical restrictions to understand that the limitations they must accept are internally rather than externally imposed constraints. If you have a medical problem, your body cannot handle certain foods. Typically, people on restricted diets react to them as if an outside authority were forbidding them certain foods. They then crave those foods which are off limits and put themselves at risk by randomly rebelling and binging on this forbidden fruit. Hard as it is to accept food restrictions of any kind, respecting your body's dictated restrictions makes it easier to live more comfortably with restraints.

It's always helpful to find out whether a restriction is absolute or whether some foods can be eaten in moderation. The more freedom you have, the easier it is to tune into exactly what you want to eat and to eat less. Even on a restricted diet, it is possible to suggest various possibilities to yourself each time you're hungry.

Q. What's the difference between watching calories and watching my hunger? Aren't you really just offering a nondiet diet?

A. It's true that when you begin to feed yourself on demand, a great deal of your energy continues to be focused on food and eating. It may very well seem to you, at the beginning, that in this respect you're no better off than you were in your dieting days. You're not measuring and counting calories, but you are giving a lot of attention to what you do with food.

We think that paying attention to your eating so you can become your own attuned feeder differs significantly from the obsessive concern about eating or not eating, which is the hallmark of all dieters. There is an important difference between obsessive and attentive thinking.

Dieters are obsessed by food and thoughts of losing weight. They are concerned about what effect each mouthful of food will have on their appearance. This weight-watching requires constant vigilance. Gain, lose, or stay the same, chronic dieters must watch their eating forever because, with all of their attempts at control, they have done nothing to change their compulsive need for food.

The craving for food can be controlled for a time by diets, but it cannot be cured by them. Although our approach to compulsive eating requires a great focus on food and eating, we are not asking you to become preoccupied with it forever. We are suggesting that you make an investment. By investing considerable attention now, you will reap rewards later. The rewards we propose are not those of a diet, temporary weight loss. You hope to lose weight permanently when you shift to demand feeding, but that weight loss will be incidental to your real victory. The most important return you can anticipate on your investment when you follow our program is the triumph over what has been an addiction.

We are offering a way out of your addiction, a permanent end to your compulsive need for food. Our goal is to get you to a point where it won't occur to you to eat unless you're hungry. Once your obsession is cured, you'll be able to have a terrible week without turning to food for comfort. We don't wish you terrible weeks, but we do want your eating life to be reliably disconnected from your emotional life and firmly connected to your real need for food.

The difference between being obsessive and being attentive merits an explanation. Dieting sets in motion a cycle that is ultimately painful and self-destructive. The attention we suggest you pay to food and eating may seem enormous at first, but as you learn to feed yourself on demand, the process becomes considerably less onerous. Once you learn what foods you need to have on hand, for example, you'll spend less time shopping. Once you learn to recognize your hunger signals, you'll spend less energy attempting to tune them in. Indeed, the attention you pay to eating will become an integral, pleasant part of your life.

Q. When I eat from mouth hunger, isn't it like going off a diet? What's the difference between feeling bad because you can't stay on a diet and feeling bad because you can't consistently feed yourself on demand?

A. Until now you've always been either on or off a diet. It makes sense that you would begin to think about demand feeding as just another diet, but it's not. It is not an outside regimen you impose on yourself; it is a response to your unique, unfolding food needs and schedule. If, after you've been eating from stomach hunger for a while, you notice that you're starting to eat from mouth hunger, it doesn't mean that you've "gone off" demand feeding. It just means that your need to eat from mouth hunger is reasserting itself and interfering with your natural pattern of eating.

You are learning to connect the sensation of hunger with food. Sometimes you do this well and accurately; at other times your need to use food for different purposes resurfaces. When it does, you notice it and can be sympathetic. Rather than scold yourself, as you would if you went off a diet, you try to learn something about the cause of your difficulty. If you're having an extended stretch of mouth hunger experiences, you ride with them patiently. The issue isn't going off or getting back on a diet. Quite the contrary.

Your problem is that you've been a mouth hunger or compulsive eater for many years. Your compulsion will gradually give way as demand feeding becomes the established way you feed yourself. You are creating a new system out of the old. That's very different from trying to get rid of or control something.

Think of it this way. Each time you feed yourself exactly what you want and as much as you need when you are hungry, you are making a deposit in a savings account labeled GOOD CARETAKING. These deposits will remain in the bank forever, and you will feel more secure as their sum grows. They are a foundation that no one and nothing can take away. When you eat from mouth hunger, your savings account is not depleted; you haven't "blown" anything. Eating from mouth hunger is simply analogous to not making a deposit. You'll get back to your deposits in due time, but even when you neglect them, your foundation remains. Patience and kindness will do the trick.

The Plan
Phase 3

Finding Yourself

– 14 –

The Compulsive
Reach for Food

When you began reading this book, you probably thought
your need to eat compulsively was evidence of greed and a
lack of willpower. You believed that your eating was a symptom of self-destructiveness. We discussed your eating in an
entirely different context, calling it a rebellion against cultural standards. And, most important, we said that when
you reached for food you were attempting to help yourself.

There was little more we could do at that point other than
alert you to how you used food and urge you to be sympathetic to rather than condemning of your need to eat. Now
you are in a position to do more.

Before you began to eat on demand, your eating was a
global response to all kinds of discomfort. Now that the
checks in your ledger have begun to move to the stomach
hunger column, you are in a position to give special consid-
eration to those times when you do eat from mouth hunger.
Remember, learning to feed yourself on demand is a gradual
process. As you nudge yourself in the direction of stomach
hunger, your desire to eat when you are not hungry will
continue to assert itself, although a lot less frequently.
Mouth hunger becomes the exception, rather than the rule,
and as such, it takes on significance.

At this point, you are ready to recognize mouth hunger as

a signal. Each time you eat out of mouth hunger you can assume that something is up, that something is making you uncomfortable. In the past, eating compulsively, then scolding yourself for it, was the ritual you employed to deal with discomfort. Some people bite their nails when they're uncomfortable, others go to sleep. You ate.

Earlier, we discussed compulsive eating as a way of coping with discomfort by translating complex concerns into an obsessive preoccupation with eating and weight. We will now examine the ritual of compulsive eating in greater detail in an effort to help you use your compulsive reach toward food as a way to better understand yourself. This ritual has two parts, a compulsive act and an obsessive thought. You reach out for food, which you have invested with magical powers, then yell at yourself for having eaten. You thereby circumvent the original source of your anxiety and relabel it "fat."

Fat Thoughts

You have spent a lifetime eating and calling yourself fat. In so doing, you have been translating your real concerns into fat concerns. You are now ready to begin decoding. First, let's review the process of translation.

You're not hungry but feel compelled to reach for food, and you eat. A few minutes—or a few hours or a few pounds—later, you are obsessed by a series of painful albeit familiar thoughts about your body and your weight and how bad you are for having eaten. These thoughts, which we call "fat thoughts," are so pervasive that compulsive eaters often have them even when they haven't eaten—in the middle of a pleasant walk, for instance.

If we were to ask you to identify your problem at the moment your fat thought strikes or right after you've eaten compulsively, you'd say something like "It's my eating. I just can't get it under control" or "It's my weight. I just don't know what I'm going to do about it." Indeed, you'd be telling us the truth as you experience it, but in translation. To the extent that you are not leveling with yourself, you would also not be leveling with us. Everytime you say "I'm fat" or "I eat too much," you are really referring to something else that you feel bad about. Compulsive eaters have many problems that they are unable to sit with or talk about in their own terms. Instead, they eat through their difficulties and say that their problem is fat. A fat thought is never about fat. It is always about an issue that got lost when you reached for food.

Of course, most people who eat compulsively and have fat thoughts are absolutely certain that their problem is eating and fat. The tenacity with which they hang on to this belief is testimony to the effectiveness of the process of translation. Once they've eaten and begun to feel bad about themselves, they no longer remember where the trouble started. They don't know that they've switched tongues, from feeling language to fat language. They know only that they feel fat and want to be rid of it.

Understanding the phenomenon of fat thoughts is complicated by the fact that some people who have them are considered by the culture to be fat. When they say "My problem is that I'm fat," their judgment is confirmed by everyone and everything around them. However, although this cultural judgment is always there, the personal fat thoughts aren't. They occur only at specific times. Why at these times and not all the time? Because fat thoughts don't concern fat. Compulsive eaters use them as a way to comment on other issues.

Lois decided to go to her twentieth high school reunion. As the date approached she noticed that she was eating more and feeling very fat. She yelled at herself for not watching her weight with such a big event on the horizon. The yelling ended with a threat—"If you don't get a grip on your eating everyone will see how fat you've become." As the reunion neared, Lois began to have second thoughts about going. In her mind, the problem was fat.

Lois's compulsive eating and weight gain might appear to be her problem. She had a history of dieting and binging, and her weight, a few weeks before the reunion, was somewhat higher than usual. However, Lois had spent a lot of time over the past few years learning how to look her best whatever her weight. Although she wished to be thinner, she was able most of the time to accept her size and was often pleased with the way she looked.

If you were to look a bit deeper at what was going on in Lois's life you'd discover that Lois was not a popular girl in high school. She had excellent grades, which made her a favorite among her teachers, but she was regarded as a square by her peers and always felt out of it socially. After high school she went to college and graduate school, where she matured socially. Lois grew up to be a well-liked adult who was quite successful in her profession.

The reunion excited Lois. She was, after all, very different from the person she'd been twenty years earlier, and she was pleased with the difference. She was eager for those who used to make fun of her to see how she had made it and to see what had become of them.

Although Lois was aware of wanting to show off at the reunion, she was unaware of the extent of her competitive feelings and her guilt about having those feelings. Rather than acknowledge and explore her discomfort, she ate, felt bad about her eating, and called herself fat. Her fat thoughts were not about fat but a condemnation of the angry feelings she had in the past and punishment for her wish to show off and retaliate for those old hurts. Lois couldn't accept these impulses within herself. In a sense, she found it easier to consider herself fat and bad than to confront her real desires.

The feelings that Lois translated into fat are, of course, specific to her. Each of us has specific issues that lead us to food and culminate in a resounding "I'm fat!"

Reaching Out for Food

The ritual of the compulsive eater begins with a reach for food. You have probably been mystified by your need to seek food when you are not the least bit hungry. When mouth hunger hits, you feel that you *have to* eat. If that means running to the freezer and eating ice cream, you do it. If it means getting into the car at midnight and searching for an all-night grocery, you're off. The urgency you feel at these moments tells us that you perceive yourself to be in danger. You don't think of it in those terms, but your actions tell a different story. You must get to the food *or else*.

Or else what? Compulsive eaters don't hang around to ask or answer that question; they run for food *before* they can think about whether they have a problem. But we do ask "Or else what?"—and we have some thoughts that you can check out against your own experience.

Each time you reach for food when you are not hungry it is because a thought or a feeling, of which you may or may not be aware, is threatening to make you anxious. You may not *feel* anxious. You run to food to ward off both the anxiety and the thought or feeling that is promoting it.

The notion that a thought or feeling could be dangerous may sound strange at first. In reality, very little could be dangerous about an idea, a wish, or an emotion. But mental life does not always adhere to the dictates of reality or logic. Indeed, in our mental lives, we are subject to fears and inhibitions that belong more to our histories than to our present-day lives. And those histories continue to shape our behavior throughout our lives.

We often attempt to avoid concerns we are not even aware of having. Think of it as being afraid of being afraid. There are a number of reasons why we attempt to avoid certain thoughts and feelings: they may fall short of our ideals, they may feel forbidden, or they may seem too strong.

Less Than Ideal: Each of us has an investment in maintaining a particular self-image. We'd prefer to strike from the record those thoughts and feelings which run counter to our ideas about who we are. It makes us anxious to think of ourselves as not living up to our ideals. It's hard, for example, for someone who thinks of herself as a very giving person to acknowledge, or even notice, that she's grown to resent her friends' calling her for advice all the time. If she's a compulsive eater, the chances are that she'll run for ice cream when she gets off the phone in preference to owning up to feelings of resentment, rethinking the responsibilities of friendship, or reformulating her responsibility to find time for herself.

Similarly, a straight-A student who has applied to top graduate schools may end up in the kitchen with his first rejection letter in one hand and a spoon in the other. It can be hard to maintain your self-esteem when faced with an unexpected rejection. Instead of experiencing the letdown and dealing with the possibility that your expectations of yourself are unrealistic or that circumstance has simply prevented you from having something you want, you eat.

Forbidden Feelings: Another source of our discomfort with thoughts and feelings has to do with notions we developed as children about the power of our wishes. For children, a wish is equivalent to a deed, a thought equivalent to an action. Since children are completely dependent on their families for survival, they are careful to think and act in ways that will ensure continued nurturing and love. A child who gets angry and says "I hate you, Mommy. I wish you were dead" is relieved to see that Mommy neither dies nor retaliates by withdrawing her love.

Although as adults we no longer depend on the good will of those around us for our survival, we often slip into the dependent mind-set of our childhood and act as though we do. Equating our thoughts with deeds, we inhibit the bad ones. Some compulsive eaters fear the forbidden emotion of anger, others fear lust, and still others fear jealousy. The list is as endless as the variety of emotions one can feel. What's important is that, as adults, we continue to fear what we consider to be unacceptable thoughts, feelings, and wishes, and we compulsive eaters attempt to erase these thoughts with food before we even know that we have them.

Laurie was furious with Mike, her boyfriend, for canceling a date at the last minute. She got off the phone and opened the fridge. As she began to eat, she thought about the movie they were supposed to have seen. She'd been looking forward to it all week. This wasn't the first time Mike had canceled at the last minute. She was furious . . . and she was emptying her refrigerator of leftovers.

Laurie had been feeding herself on demand for a few months, so she noticed immediately when she began eating from mouth hunger. She knew that it was important to allow herself to eat without shouting, and she tried to think about why she was turning to food when she wasn't really hungry. "What just happened?" she asked herself. "I got off the phone feeling furious. I can't stand being stood up this way. I'd really like to throw the refrigerator at Mike. But I didn't even say a word to him about how angry and disappointed I am. I was nice to him on the phone, the good little girl I was raised to be. My mother told me to be polite, and here I am. When I was a kid I feared the wrath of God and the church. Now I act as though Mike will excommunicate me just because I'm angry. Well, even if I'm afraid to say anything to Mike, I have to get more comfortable with my anger so I don't keep reaching for food. When I try to eat my anger away it just smolders until the next eruption."

Strong Feelings: Some of us are less concerned with the permissibility of our thoughts and feelings than with the issue of their intensity, fearing that we will somehow be overwhelmed by our inner lives. People who have this fear say things like "If I let myself feel sad, I'll never stop being depressed" or "If I get angry, I'll go out of control." These people do not understand that feelings are transient and use food to keep themselves on an even keel.

Interestingly, some compulsive eaters fear not only the intensity of their feelings, but any change in the status quo. For them, any strong feeling or change results in the reach for food. The implication is that they see themselves as fragile and in need of a carefully controlled atmosphere.

Carol remembered during a workshop that whenever something bothered her as a child, her parents urged her not to get so upset. She realized that whenever her feelings threaten to become slightly intense, she runs for food. Months after this realization she happened to be talking to her mother, describing her struggle with a difficult situation at work. Her mother's immediate response was "Don't get too upset about it," and this time it made Carol laugh. "Why shouldn't I get upset? It's an upsetting situation," she said. Much to her surprise, her mother caught on and responded, "You know, you're right. You have every reason to be upset and I hope things will get better soon."

Of course, most compulsive eaters are aware of the futility of reaching for food when they're in distress, yet they continue to do so. This is not a logical act. They reach for food because they invest it with magical powers.

Making Food into Magic

A New York bakery sells a brownie called "Magic Mommie." These bakers have an intuitive understanding of the symbolic power food holds for compulsive eaters. Compulsive eaters believe in food the way we all once believed that our parents were endowed with the magical power to solve all our problems. Food represents many things to compulsive eaters—mother, father, family, love, safety, strength, comfort, power, support, and on and on.

When we feel desperate and turn to food, it is as if we expect to take in all that it symbolizes as well. For compulsive eaters food is the centerpiece of a ritual to ward off danger. For the compulsive eater, eating in response to danger is no different than standing on one foot and hopping in a circle once to the right and twice to the left might have been for a member of a primitive tribe who felt threatened by a clap of thunder. The ritual feels essential.

It's helpful to look at some of the magical expectations compulsive eaters have of food.

Teddy Bears: Anyone who has noticed a toddler dragging a blanket around or clutching a teddy bear to his breast understands the power of symbols. Symbolically, that teddy is very much alive to its owner. If you leave it behind when you go away for a weekend you pay dearly. At the height of his power, Teddy represents all the care and support that its owner has known. With Teddy around she can be sure she is safe. Once she is able to ensure her own well-being, however, she no longer needs the magic of Teddy. With its symbolic power gone, the same bear will end up, neglected, in a heap of toys.

As symbol-making creatures, we invest all kinds of objects—bears, rabbits' feet, prayers, chants, leaders, and, *food*—with the power to make us feel safe. Sadly, the efficacy of food is not the same as that of a teddy. Teddy bears and other transitional objects, so named by British psychoanalyst D. W. Winnicott, help toddlers feel more secure for as long as they use them. When they outlive their usefulness, however, they are quickly discarded. In the sense that teddy bears are instrumental in moving children from one stage to the next, they work. Food doesn't.

Teddy bears have no function other than to soothe. Food does. The primary function of food is nourishment. When food is used for comfort, its proper function is neglected entirely and it becomes addicting instead of enabling. We suggest that you carry food around with you not as a teddy bear, but so you can feel secure in the knowledge that whenever you're hungry you will be fed. When you feel fed and well cared for, you'll no longer need to use food as a teddy bear.

Whiteout: Another of our expectations of food goes far beyond our need for comfort and addresses our desire to eradicate problems. To that end, compulsive eaters use food the way a typist uses whiteout. When a typist makes an error, something appears on the printed page that doesn't belong there. Whiteout covers the error and gives the page the appearance of being perfect. When you hold the paper up to the light, however, you can still see the typo behind the brush strokes of the correcting fluid, and therein lies the critical difference between everything's being all right and everything's appearing to be all right.

Using food as a temporary patch to cover underlying problems does nothing to address them. For the moment its magic lasts, food feels soothing to the compulsive eater. Eating is, after all, a pleasurable activity, and the pleasure allows us momentarily to sidestep our pain. Unfortunately, the pleasure of food is fleeting. It may fill us up, symbolically and literally, but its capacity to soothe is flawed. Ultimately, food eaten compulsively is nothing more than a distractor that functions as a link between one kind of distress and another.

When we eat compulsively, we switch our focus from the food to our feeling of physical discomfort. It's hard to think about much else when you feel stuffed, and when the stuffed feeling passes, your distress shifts from physical to mental discomfort. You think about the consequences of eating and latch onto a series of negative, painful thoughts about yourself—your eating, your body, and the hopelessly degraded state of your character.

In the past you opted for these painful thoughts instead of identifying your real problems. On one level that strategy made sense. If the problem were truly a fat problem you could diet it away. People are often quite reluctant to give up mislabeling their problems "fat."

Joan told us that she'd been eating out of mouth hunger quite a bit and couldn't stop yelling at herself for it. We discovered that her brother had visited her for the weekend and her out-of-control eating seemed to be related to that event. When she was asked about her relationship to her brother, it became clear to everyone in the group that Joan's ambivalent feelings toward him were strikingly intense and that her problem was certainly not her fat. As one woman put it, "I can see why Joan would rather yell at herself for eating. It's really a lot easier to feel bad about being fat than it is to face up to feelings you've always been told you shouldn't have. At least you can get rid of fat. What are you going to do about your anger at your brother and the guilt it induces?"

While it is true that superficially it may seem easier to deal with fat than with hostility, which you feel guilty about, calling your problem "fat" is, in the long run, a dead-end strategy for coping. You feel justly punished as a result of your self-rebuke but remain stuck. Hopefully, as you begin to see the futility of attempting to diet such problems away, you will be able to intervene when you start to translate your concerns in this way.

The Implications of Making Food into Magic

The truth is that once an idea, wish, or feeling exists in mental life, it remains there. You can think about it, you can act on it, you can decide not to act on it, you can find an alternative way of expressing it, or you can attempt to deny its existence—white it out. But when you attempt to deny that something exists it reappears in a different shape—in the shape of "fat thoughts." You can't get very far away from the fact that something is bothering you.

When we reach for food before we know what's bothering us, we are responding automatically, based on some old assumptions. When we reach before we even ask if we're hungry, we're assuming that we're not up to dealing with much, and we're probably selling ourselves short.

Throughout this book we have said that you should continue to eat from mouth hunger until you no longer feel the need to and that before you can begin to feel more grounded and secure, you will probably need a lot of attuned eating experiences. We're not suggesting otherwise at this point. It's important to understand, however, that anxiety is a signal, a warning that something is brewing. When we eat from mouth hunger we are dousing that signal with food, consequently depriving ourselves of the opportunity to learn something about ourselves that may help us in the future. If we allow ourselves to feel the anxiety, we stand a chance of becoming aware of our problems and giving them names, the first step toward effective problem solving.

Gary took a three-week vacation from his highly stressful job and went off to New Mexico. Before he left on the trip his eating had been more or less out of stomach hunger. During the last week of his vacation, however, he noticed that he was popping jelly beans into his mouth every few minutes, eating more out of mouth hunger than stomach hunger, and he was beginning to feel heavier. Gary was distressed about his weight, but before he allowed himself to slip into his old pattern of yelling, he stopped himself. He knew that something had to have been making him anxious. The question was "What?"

"It's been a great vacation," he thought, "but this eating must be a sign that something is wrong." Gary tried to figure out what his problem was, and it didn't take long for him to make some headway in his investigation.

He realized that he had begun to eat from mouth hunger ten days earlier, just after he had checked in with his office. When Gary had left on his vacation, he was filled with dread about the problems he was leaving behind and what he'd have to confront when he returned. His call home confirmed his worst fears. There was no question about how desperately he'd needed to get away, but he'd be returning to a mammoth mess.

Once Gary named his anxiety "returning to the office," he stopped eating about it and went back to eating from stomach hunger. Gary continued to feel anxious from time to time during the last week of his vacation, but he tried to use his anxiety as a signal to take a few moments and think about one of his upcoming problems.

The value of developing an awareness of what is causing you discomfort is that you can look at it with a clear head in the light of day. You can ask yourself a few questions. Is what I'm thinking really so terrible? Is what I'm feeling so reprehensible? Can I let myself feel what I'm feeling and know that the feeling will pass? Can I think through a solution to my dilemma? Maybe I can just forget about what's bothering me and space out for a while.

All problems require a good deal of thought and individually tailored solutions. Eating offers precisely the opposite. It inhibits thought and treats all problems as if they were the same, homogenizing them. The more you eat on demand, the more possible it will be for you to look at, rather than eat around, some of your real concerns.

People who use this approach primarily feel a tremendous relief about breaking their addiction to food. There are, however, additional rewards. Once you no longer need to reach compulsively for food, you have the opportunity to discover your real concerns and have the energy with which to address them. Before you can do that, however, you have to address the finale of the ritual of compulsive eating, your obsessive thoughts about eating and your body.

– 15 –

The Obsession

What Is All the Yelling About?

The sequence begins with discomfort. Some thought, situation, or feeling is producing anxiety and you are aware only that you want to eat. The sequence ends with the discomfort that comes from scolding yourself and calling yourself names. You feel just as compelled to shout at yourself after you have eaten as you do to eat in the first place. Yelling at yourself completes the circuit—it ends the ritual.

The point of compulsive eating is ostensibly to put an end to your discomfort. The obsessive thoughts about fat that necessarily follow from your eating, however, long outlast any fleeting comfort that comes from food. Many of you spend much of your free time ruminating about your eating and your weight, about your unacceptability. The words "I'm fat" or "I eat too much" are the mantras of compulsive eaters. The point of a mantra for meditation is to fill your mind with one word, thereby clearing it of all other concerns. Once the mantra is in place, you can begin to feel inner peace.

The problem with using "I'm fat" or "I eat too much" as a mantra is that although it may push other concerns out of your mind, it doesn't bring you inner peace. Instead, it fills your mind with pain. "I'm fat, I'm fat, I'm fat" means "I'm bad, I'm bad, I'm bad."

I'm Bad . . .

We hope we've convinced you by now that fat thoughts are never about fat. The time has come to try to figure out what they *are* about.

Generally, when compulsive eaters yell at themselves about being fat they are shouting about either their need for help, in the shape of food, to deal with their anxiety or about whatever feeling sent them to food in the first place.

Because I Shouldn't Need Help: We have spoken about food as a symbol of earlier caretaking, and the reach for food as a reach back in time for comfort. Sadly, many compulsive eaters who take this route condemn themselves for needing to take it, and their condemnation takes the form of yelling and fat thoughts. They become, in a sense, their own angry parent. "When are you going to grow up?" they seem to be saying. "When are you going to be able to stand up on your own two feet and stop running home for help?"

The impulse to reach back to food for help and then scold yourself is complicated by the fact that every compulsive eater knows that the food is not going to help and will make things more difficult. As a result, they consider themselves stupid and ridiculous and can't forgive themselves for needing to run home.

Amanda, a competent director of a mental health center, is known for her leadership and organizational skills. Everyone she works with knows that if they want something done, Amanda is the one to do it.

On the surface, Amanda appears to have made it. She commands a high salary, has a beautiful home and lots of good friends, but she is miserable because she is overweight.

As she describes it, "I can't stand it anymore. Why do I have to eat this way? I'm getting bigger and bigger. I have to get my eating in control. I'm really in shock that I've let myself go like this. I would love to be more accepting about my need to eat, but I just can't be. It's a terrible embarrassment to me that I look like this, that I can't deal with the whole problem."

Amanda clearly hates feeling out of control. Her need to use food when she's in emotional difficulty drives her nuts. She prides herself on being self-sufficient, on not having to turn to others for help, and she takes her need for food when she's in trouble as a sign of weakness. It makes her angry. The self-contempt she focuses on fat is really caused by her perception of herself as weak if she needs help.

What can Amanda and people like her do about feeling that they are deficient because they cannot make it through a problem without turning to food? We agree that it would be much better if no one had to use food in a driven, addicted way. That's why we've written this book. But it's critical to keep in mind that your turning to food is not a moral issue. It simply is. As you really care for yourself and eat out of stomach hunger, you'll have less need for the symbolic care that mouth hunger offers. If, on the other hand, you continue to scold yourself for eating, you will have to eat more to comfort yourself. More important, you will be closing the circuit and enabling the ritual of compulsive eating to work. Each time you close the circuit by scolding yourself, you make it more difficult to find out what sent you to food.

Because I Have Bad Thoughts and Feelings: When you say "I'm bad for eating," the chances are that what you mean is "I'm bad for feeling or thinking what I was about to feel or think before I ate." You've made the translation from a feeling that made you anxious to a fat thought, but the source of your concern is still alive inside. You've just displaced the sense of badness from your feeling to your fat.

Amy was asked by Lily, her closest friend, for a favor. Lily had an important business dinner coming up on a Friday night and couldn't find a baby-sitter. Amy loved Lily's children and had often baby-sat for them in the past. This time, however, it really wasn't convenient. Amy had already made plans of her own for that night and was looking forward to them. Rather than say that she couldn't help, however, Amy said, "Gee, I'd love to do it but I have tentative plans." Then Amy thought to herself, "I might be able to cancel them, but I'm so tired by the end of the week that I really need to look forward to something pleasant. I've been feeling depressed and I think that if I don't go out with my friends on Friday I'll probably feel bad."

Later in the week, Lily, not having found a sitter, called to inquire about Amy's plans. Amy felt guilty about not offering to cancel her engagement, but she decided to hold her ground and told Lily that she wouldn't be able to help. Lily didn't say anything directly, but Amy knew she was hurt. They went back a long way and this kind of thing had come up before. Although Amy usually did what she thought was right, she rarely took her own needs into account. This time she did.

A few hours after the last conversation with Lily, Amy confirmed her own plans for Friday and started eating chocolate-covered almonds. She knew she wasn't hungry, but she had to eat them. Her mind flashed to the conversation with Lily. She could almost hear the disappointment and the slight disapproval in Lily's voice. It made Amy anxious just thinking about it. She felt bad for not helping out—selfish, not nice—and she kept eating the almonds. In the past, she would have started berating herself for eating them. This time she was able to think about her dilemma rather than tie it up in a fat package. As she struggled to think, instead of feeling fat, she realized how anxious she gets when she has to say no to people she's close to. She feels mean when she does it and is sure they'll be angry if she doesn't accommodate them. It wasn't easy for Amy to live with the feeling of having done a "bad" thing. In spite of her anxiety, however, she actually felt stronger for having been able to say no.

Amy will continue to have conflicts about what she thinks is good and bad. Now that she recognizes that it's not her fat or eating that she feels bad about, she is in a position to struggle with her real problem, her inability to say no comfortably.

Breaking the Circuit

We have spoken throughout this book about the importance of accepting your need to eat. When you understand how your obsessive thoughts about eating and weight obscure the issues that send you to food, you can see how vital it is to stop translating feelings into fat thoughts. When your energy is bound up in self-contempt, you run head-on into two problems—you lose sight of the real problem, and should you gain sight of it, you have no energy left for problem solving.

Unlike your compulsion to eat, which will fade as you feed yourself differently and treat yourself with compassion, your compulsion to yell at yourself requires direct intervention. Once compulsive eaters understand how they move from compulsive eating to obsessive thinking, we urge them to stop making the translation. We call this "breaking the circuit."

When you eat from mouth hunger, you eat because you must. When your mind starts moving in the direction of self-condemnation, however, you have an opportunity to intervene. You can break the addictive circuit in two ways:

1. Remind yourself each time you eat from mouth hunger that you will not scold yourself after you eat.
2. Never take a fat thought at face value. Each time you find yourself shouting at yourself for eating or being fat, remind yourself that you are referring to something else and, if you can, make an effort to find out what that something else is.

You will discover that breaking the circuit is easier said than done. You want to close the circuit by yelling at yourself. The pull to do so often feels irresistible. What is so compelling about all the yelling?

Why the Yelling Is Compelling: You've been involved in the ritual of compulsive eating for many years and berating yourself is an essential part of it. Your reasons for holding on to fat thoughts are, on one level, quite compelling. First of all, life is much simpler when all roads lead to one destination. If all of your problems can be reduced to an eating problem, you needn't look further than one solution for them—diet. If you stop yelling, you break the circuit and stop translating all problems into fat. Faced with myriad problems you'll need to come up with solutions, and that isn't easy.

Second, life is scarier when you stop translating all problems into fat. It was, after all, a fear of your real problems that led you to translate them into fat in the first place. Breaking the circuit will put you face to face with whatever you were trying to escape. This confrontation is not a pleasant prospect.

Third, you've grown accustomed to your yelling. Although yelling at yourself is painful, for many it's the only way you know to be with yourself. In a strange way, it's comforting. Attempt to separate a child from an abusive parent and, more often than not, he will resist. That parent is the only parent he knows. It's a loss, but sometimes it feels better to be yelled at than not to get any attention at all.

Finally, when you eat in response to forbidden feelings, your yelling serves as a punishment for those feelings and simultaneously keeps them alive. If you say "I feel angry" in a neutral, observing voice, you defuse the anger. If, instead, you translate your angry feeling into the reach for food, then berate yourself for being fat and disgusting, the drama of your angry feeling remains charged. If you don't do something you would like to do because you question its moral correctness or are concerned about hurting someone you care about, you are choosing self-respect and freedom from guilt over doing what you want. If you then feel frustrated or disappointed, eat, and yell at yourself, you'll be keeping the original situation alive by eating what seems to you to be forbidden fruit and scolding yourself for it.

However, despite all these compelling reasons to yell, there are more compelling reasons to stop. Primary among them is the emergence of your "self," with all its quirks and complications. As we've said throughout, you are much more interesting and complex than fat, and you'll need all of the energy you've been pouring into your yelling to come to grips with who you are.

The Emergence of a Complex Self: If you feed yourself on demand and stop yelling at yourself about fat and eating, you will probably discover that you are entirely able to face anxiety and give your problems their proper names. All this, of course, happens gradually, and it follows a course.

Think about your potential progress in the following stages:

1. You reach for food when you're not hungry as a stock response to a wide variety of problems.
2. You eat from stomach hunger much of the time and from mouth hunger in response to anxiety that stems from problems you're unable to name or confront.
3. You have the impulse to eat from mouth hunger but use it as a signal of anxiety instead. You spot it and are able to say "Aha! What's going on? What am I anxious about?"
4. You experience anxiety, just like everybody else! Maybe you're a little more savvy than most and can use it as a signal that something is brewing and needs your attention.

Barbara is a compulsive eater who kept working at breaking the circuit. She left work at 5:00 P.M. after a good day at the office. She strolled home feeling quite pleased with herself. At some point she noticed a couple walking arm in arm in the opposite direction, engaged in deep conversation. As they passed Barbara, her mood changed almost imperceptibly. She stopped in front of a doughnut shop and began to think about the doughnuts in the window. She noticed that she was not really hungry. "This must be mouth hunger," she said to herself.

Before Barbara entered the doughnut shop she had the following internal dialogue. "I've been doing so well with feeding myself on demand, I don't want to ruin it now with these doughnuts. I really shouldn't. Wait a minute, that's the old diet voice speaking. Yes, I am doing well with feeding my stomach hunger. Since I'm not hungry now, I wonder what's making me want a doughnut. I wasn't upset when I left the office; I was feeling really good. Do I need doughnuts now or can I wait until my stomach is hungry?" Barbara paused. "I need them now and I'm going to have them. I know that the best way to help myself is to buy a huge supply of my favorite doughnuts. I just have to remember not to yell at myself later."

Ordering a dozen glazed doughnuts, Barbara ate two in the store and another on the street. She knew that she was eating more than she wanted but tried to go with it. She felt good having the supply of doughnuts with her. Once home, Barbara took another doughnut, ate half of it, and put what was left of the doughnuts in the freezer. They belong to her. She can have them whenever she's mouth or stomach hungry.

Later in the evening she remembered the episode and tried to understand what happened. "I was feeling good when I left the office, so what happened on my way home? I remember that I noticed a handsome-looking couple walk by me. It's hard to believe that they set me off, but it's the first thing that comes to mind. I certainly noticed them. I think that I thought they looked happy and involved with each other. I guess I felt envious and lonely. It was soon after I passed them that I noticed the doughnut shop. I guess I just didn't want to deal with feeling envious and alone. I'll have to watch to see if those feelings often trigger my desire to eat."

Barbara broke the addictive circuit. She ate but she didn't berate herself, and later she was able to figure out what had troubled her. She achieved a victory in dealing with her mouth hunger this way. By eating three and a half doughnuts instead of polishing them all off in a few hours, she learned about possible psychological triggers for her eating and avoided an evening of self-hate and recrimination. By being sympathetic about her need to eat and feeding herself on demand, Barbara will get to a point where she'll be able to see a couple walk by and experience her feelings of loneliness and envy without turning to doughnuts.

A few days later when Barbara found herself standing in front of her freezer door, face to face with her doughnuts, she recognized that she was not hungry and thought back to the last few minutes before her trip to the refrigerator. She had just ended a phone conversation with one of her closest friends, who had called to say "Guess what? I'm pregnant." Barbara was genuinely thrilled for her friend, who had had a difficult time conceiving. But there was no doubt that the phone call had brought her to the freezer door. Barbara closed the door and analyzed her feelings. "I'd love to have a child," she thought. "I wish I didn't feel so envious of my friends' lives." This expressed, Barbara went into the living room, cried a little, and turned on the TV. She soon became absorbed in the program.

Barbara has come a long way. She is able to use her desire to reach for food as a signal that she must pay attention to her feelings. She has stopped translating her concerns into fat thoughts and is consequently more comfortable and realistic about herself and her life. She may have many problems to solve, but by labeling them correctly, she'll be in a better position to work at them more effectively.

– 16 –

When You Try to
Break the Circuit

Once you understand the dynamics involved in your compulsion to eat and your obsession with fat, you have a solid basis from which to make a meaningful change. As is always the case, however, there's a significant difference between understanding something in your head and applying that understanding to your life. That difference is best explored by examining the questions people ask as they attempt to stop translating and start breaking the addictive circuit of compulsive eating.

Q. If it's true that for years I've been eating to avoid problems that make me anxious, how do I know that I can handle not avoiding them. How do I know that I'm up to facing the things that drive me to eat? Won't I be overwhelmed by anxiety?

A. We said earlier that many compulsive eaters are afraid to stop eating and yelling because they don't know what they'll have to face once they do. This question reflects that very real fear.

Your calling a problem fat doesn't mean that you've done anything about the problem. It simply means that you have named it incorrectly. If you call your envy "fat," you will continue to have a problem with envy. If you call your sadness "fat," you will continue to have a problem with sadness. If, however, you acknowledge the envy or sadness, allowing yourself to feel them in their untranslated state, you have a chance to examine these emotions. And therein lies the possibility of meaningful relief.

It's also important to understand that even if you don't name your real problems, you continue to suffer from them. The pain of yelling at yourself, of wincing when you see yourself in the mirror, of never feeling good about the way you look, is every bit as painful as the real problem that drives you to food. It's the same pain with a different facade. You've coped with it until now, and you'll cope with it when you know what it's about, either on your own or with help.

Ginny felt a great deal of pain when she stopped her usual shouting. She was in the middle of a bad divorce and felt terribly anxious. She had been eating compulsively, and when she stopped scolding herself about it, the anger that she customarily leveled at herself was replaced by a profound sadness; her handling of that sadness is interesting— she took it to bed. Whereas in the past she would have eaten and experienced her sadness as yelling, she now felt her sadness and retreated to bed, where she stayed until she felt some relief.

"Retreating to my bed when I feel overwhelmed by my sadness makes more sense to me than eating and screaming," Ginny explained. "I don't like being upset and nonfunctional, and sometimes I have to eat first and then go to bed, but during this period I've really thought a lot about why I'm so unhappy. I'm grappling with things so much more complicated than my weight, which was the focus of all my thoughts until I stopped yelling at myself for eating. I remembered last night that during the year after my father died I gained lots of weight. I realize now that I never really dealt with the loss. Instead, I kept thinking I had a weight problem. My divorce stirs up the same feelings of loss. I may have to get some help with them, but at least I'll be dealing with real loss, not weight loss."

You have no way to know in advance what your experience will be when you stop mislabeling your problems. We believe that you will feel infinitely better, and considerably less anxious, once you start feeding yourself on demand and treating yourself well. We cannot know, however, what particular problem you have been eating about.

Compulsive eaters all approach problems in the same way. They all believe that they cannot calm themselves without running to food. The problems they approach, however, vary as do their fears about what will happen if they don't use food to calm down.

Should you find that demand feeding does not lessen your anxiety and calm you down enough to begin thinking about your problems, you may need outside help, psychotherapy or counseling. If that turns out to be the case, it means that you, like Ginny, will seek help for what's bothering you rather than for your weight, and that is a great advance.

Q. If I don't reach for food when I experience mouth hunger, what should I do instead? Distract myself? Take a bath? Do something nice for myself?

A. Compulsive eaters often fall into the "feel-something-do-something trap." They imagine that if they don't eat and call themselves fat when they're anxious, they must do something instead.

We feel very strongly about your not having to do anything with your feelings. Of course it's great if you can express your feelings and find a way to work out whatever is troubling you. But you can't always do that, and when you can't, it's appropriate to just sit with whatever is disturbing you.

There's a myth in our culture that you should do something nice for yourself when you feel bad. If you feel isolated and depressed, buy yourself a hat or run a bubble bath. You'll emerge feeling like a new person. The reality is that we don't always feel like pampering ourselves when we're upset. Sometimes doing something pleasurable does improve our mood, but it's not always possible to handle bad feelings this way.

You may wonder what a noncompulsive eater does instead of turning to food when she or he is anxious. It depends entirely on who that noncompulsive eater is. Many people attempt to bypass their feelings in ways other than eating—they drink, they develop somatic symptoms, or use other compulsive activities. Many noncompulsive people, however, have a more varied repertoire. They name their feelings; they feel them; they think about them; they decide to act on them; they decide not to act on them; they simply accept what they're feeling until it passes; or they often just forget about what they're thinking or feeling.

Ideally, at some point you will be able to regard mouth hunger as a signal that something is wrong. If you're inclined to, you may be able to figure out what the something is, and figuring it out may be all that's necessary.

Claire is a perfect example of someone who has learned to use the signal of mouth hunger as a red alert. "I went to the supermarket to do my weekly shopping," Claire explained. "When I headed for the checkout counter a woman with a wagon filled to the brim jumped in front of me. I was furious, but I didn't say anything. I stood there feeling that she had shoved me out of the way, watching as the cashier began to ring up her mountain of food. After a minute or so I reached into my own cart and came up with a bag of Fritos. As I did it I asked myself, 'Why am I eating? I'm not the least bit hungry.' I've gotten to a point where I understand that eating when I'm not hungry is just my way of saying I'm anxious. So I backtracked and found that, beyond my obvious rage at this woman and my frustration at not being able to say anything to her about jumping ahead of me, I was also a bit envious of her ability to do that. I ate a few Fritos, but the more I thought it out, the less interest I had in eating."

Not all compulsive eaters should expect to have Claire's sense of resolution once they figure out what their anxiety is about. Even without that resolution, however, you don't need the yelling. You can put whatever is bothering you aside.

"Last night I had the urge to eat when I wasn't hungry," Bert told us. "I noticed it and tried to figure out what was disturbing me. I'd been watching a TV movie about a guy who reacted to losing his job by drinking, so I thought back to having lost a job myself many years ago. But that didn't seem to make me anxious. I suddenly flashed back to a scene in this movie between the man and his father and then I felt the twinge. It's almost embarrassing to see that I'm so vulnerable to a grade B movie, but somehow it really touched a nerve.

"My last visit with my folks was unpleasant. I felt as though my father was grilling me about my life and I finally lost my temper. As I thought about that weekend I started to get agitated. So I stopped myself and decided to think about it some other time. Until then I didn't know that I was capable of just deciding not to think about something. It's a great discovery. I watched a little more TV, leafed through a magazine, but basically I just spaced out. Spacing out may not solve my problem but until I'm ready to do that, it sure beats eating."

Spacing out is a way to put things on hold. We don't condone it or condemn it as a way of life, but it is an option that most compulsive eaters are unaware of. It's one of many things one can do with thoughts and feelings besides eating about them.

Q. I've often known what I was feeling but eaten anyway. If I can figure out what's making me anxious, shouldn't that stop me from eating?

A. It's not unusual to know what your problem is and continue to eat. Remember, insight alone does not solve compulsive eating. You need to experience demand feeding, which is a process that takes effect in the long haul. Only gradually does taking care of yourself this way eliminate mouth hunger. Consequently, you may know what's disturbing you, but if you don't feel confident enough to really deal with it, or if you're unable to put it aside, you may very well find yourself at the refrigerator in need of support.

Go with it sympathetically and you'll soon find stomach hunger again. Your knowledge of what's bothering you is a plus. Next time you're in the same situation perhaps you'll be more comfortable with it and not have to move toward food.

Becka said, "The other morning my husband and I had a terrible fight and, predictably, I spent the rest of that day running to food. I understand that there are issues in all long-term relationships that never get completely resolved and reassert themselves periodically, but on a deeper level I still get anxious when we fight. So why I was eating wasn't a mystery to me for a minute.

"Before I began eating on demand, I would have tried to stop myself. After all, if you know what the problem is, why eat? And of course, after telling myself I *shouldn't* eat, I would have headed straight for the fridge. Now I understand that whether or not I eat from mouth hunger is not the big issue. What matters is that I stay sympathetic to myself during a crisis. I hope to get to a point where I no longer run to food when I'm anxious. Knowing what triggers my mouth hunger is part of reaching that goal, but only a part. You can *know*, but if you're not able to calm yourself, your hand will still reach for food. And the most important thing is not to dump on yourself if it does."

Q. If I stop eating compulsively, won't I develop another symptom? After all, if my problems aren't all resolved, where will the anxiety go?

A. This is a logical question. People commonly think that if you end one compulsion you take up another, trading smoking for eating, gambling for drinking, nail biting for hair twirling.

If you don't *resolve* a compulsion, if, as often happens, you attempt to free yourself of it by sheer willpower, namely, deprivation, you probably will notice that you've replaced it with a new one. If, however, you end a compulsion by treating yourself well, you won't move on to another one.

We have spoken throughout this book about the more profound implications of becoming your own demand feeder, about how you change each time you have an experience of feeding stomach hunger, and how those experiences build on each other. Although feeding yourself on demand and developing self-compassion will not solve all your problems—or eliminate all your anxiety—that sort of treatment will reassure you that an attuned caretaker is on the scene. That kind of reassurance, which you don't get when you "kick" a habit, contributes to your sense of security and makes switching compulsions unnecessary. Giving something to yourself is very different from taking something away.

Q. Two activities fill up my days—eating compulsively and yelling at myself. You've given me lots of good advice about what to do when I want to eat from mouth hunger, and you've given me stomach hunger to take its place. But what am I supposed to do when I want to yell at myself? I can't imagine not sneering at myself in the mirror. What can you offer me to replace my yelling?

A. We were intrigued by this question, so we decided to open it up to a group that had been working on the problem of their compulsive eating for some time and see how they would answer. One woman just laughed and said, "Tell people that when they give up contempt they are left with pure anxiety!" This woman has had a lifetime of experience calling herself fat and knows how difficult it is to start eating on demand and give up the self-abuse. She experienced a great deal of anxiety as she became a more attuned self-feeder, because she discovered things about herself that made her uncomfortable. She grew up with very rigid ideas about what it meant to be a "nice" person, and many of the feelings she had been eating away didn't fall into that category. As she acknowledged those feelings she felt anxious rather than just fat.

Someone else said, "You don't replace your yelling with anything except reality." Indeed, reality, with its variety of problems, is what emerges when you give up your fat thoughts. That reality is more complex and less subject to magical solutions than fat, and some people complain that reality is a letdown. They miss the intense feelings that accompany the fantasy of thinness in thirty days. Most people, however, feel considerably more relaxed without so much yelling and yearning.

"I feel that a caring, gentle new person is living in my head," one woman said. "It's as though I've been adopted by a new parent who does things very differently from the old one. She's not critical, but she's not indulgent, either. She doesn't yell if I eat when I'm not hungry, she makes sure that I've always got plenty of the foods I like, and she helps me pick out clothing I feel good about."

"I know what you mean," someone else said. "But she doesn't coddle and she's no Pollyanna. When I eat from mouth hunger, if I can't figure out what's going on, this voice inside me sees to it that I work on it the next day. And if I can wait for stomach hunger, that same voice says something kind and urges me to keep eating from stomach hunger as many times a day as possible. Basically, this new voice inside my head lets me think or feel absolutely anything—as long as I give things their proper names."

Sounds like good company to us.

– 17 –

Fat, Skinny, and In-Between

Most of you have had a painful relationship to your body for many years. We hope that, in this book, we have convinced you that your negative feelings about your body are culturally engendered and, if anything, distract you from real issues. We don't, however, expect this newfound conviction immediately to reverse a lifetime of bad feelings about your body. Indeed, it's likely that despite any new insights, you're still quite concerned about losing weight.

We understand how difficult it is for lifetime dieters to give up the part of them that has always been "weight watching." We understand that most of you are reading this book because you want to make a drastic change in the size of your body, and we are sympathetic to that wish. However, we hope you understand that we think it is impossible for you to work directly on changing your weight. You need, instead, to be compassionate and accepting of your body size while you work to end your food addiction.

This is, of course, easier said than done. Not only must you work against your own prejudices, but you must also continue to confront a world in which people insist that your well-being depends on your losing weight and that the only obstacle to weight loss is a weak character. You must be able to stand firm in the belief that diets don't work and that weight loss does not cure most ills.

As a result of breaking your addiction to food, most of you will lose weight—return to your natural, lower weight. In this chapter we will describe what happens to your weight as you become better able to feed yourself on demand.

The Reality of Weight Loss

When compulsive eaters discuss weight loss they say things like

"I really want to free myself from my obsession with food and weight, but I know that if I could just lose some weight I would feel healthier, move more easily, be less physically weighed down."

And,

"It's always been true of me that I feel much better about myself when I'm thinner. Besides, every doctor will tell you how important it is for health reasons to lose weight. Wouldn't I be better off if I lost some weight quickly and then tried your approach, to sort of give myself a head start?"

Think about the last time you lost weight quickly. How quickly did you gain it back, and how much did you regain? Statistics indicate that when people regain the weight they lose on diets they gain it plus more. There is no question but that the yo-yo effect of diets is dangerous to your psychological and physical health. As reported in the *New York Times* for March 24, 1987, Dr. George Blackburn, an obesity specialist at Harvard Medical School, stated, "At least half of obese people who try to diet down to the *desirable* weights listed in the height-weight tables suffer medically, physically and psychologically as a result, and would be better off fat."

In that same article, Jane Brody noted that new studies indicate that relatively small weight losses—10 percent of body weight—can correct a tendency toward diabetes or high blood pressure, but beyond this, claims made for thinness or against fatness have never been well substantiated.

We said that we were sympathetic to your wish to lose weight, and we are. The truth is that thin people have an easier time fitting in, finding clothing that fits well and looks attractive, and they stand a better chance socially. There's no arguing with these facts. Our point, however, is that your desire to be thinner and your determined, diligent efforts toward that end have not made you thinner. As we see it, the only chance you have to change your shape permanently is first to stand up against the cultural notion of the one acceptable body type and proceed to work on your addiction to food, which is, after all, your real problem.

Dealing with Doctors: We know how hard it is to face the fact that diets don't work. We know that dieters feel that they, not the diets, have failed. Unfortunately, those feelings of failure are usually heightened when you consult a physican. Members of the medical profession, feeling duty bound to promote thinness, often forget that no one wants to lose weight more than you, the person whose weight is above the cultural norm. Doctors talk to you as though you were unaware of the problem, as though you hadn't already devoted much of your life's energy to thoughts and strategies about weight loss. Because compulsive eaters associate doctors with this sort of attitude, many avoid seeing physicians when they should. They fear that even if they visit a doctor to obtain relief for a common cold, he or she will comment about their weight. We have a few suggestions to help you deal with this.

Remind yourself before you go to the doctor's office that

you are operating under a new set of assumptions for which you have new strategies. The doctor, like others in your life, probably lives with the accepted cultural viewpoint about fat and weight loss. He has his view, you have yours. And if you are worried about the confrontation, you might prefer to raise the issue yourself at the beginning of the consultation and voice your concern. One woman we know told her doctor that she hadn't made an appointment for many years because she dreaded the usual criticism about her weight. She told him that she, like everyone else, would love to lose weight, but that until she was able to stop eating out of anxiety it simply wasn't going to happen.

If you're not comfortable with quite so direct an approach, you can wait for the subject to come up, then say, "I'm working on losing weight as best I can. I'm sure you know that most weight lost is usually regained, and I've spent too much of my life going up and down. I'm hoping that I'll lose slowly and permanently by trying to live differently with food. In the meantime, I'm trying to live life as fully as I can the way I am."

Of course, the big question in terms of a visit to the doctor is what to do about the weigh-in, a standard procedure during most physical examinations. We have a number of suggestions. You can explain that knowing your exact weight hinders the approach you are taking to eating and request that he or she not weigh you. Or you can allow yourself to be weighed but ask not to be told the results. The important thing for you to remember is that the scale no longer has a place in your life.

When the Weight Begins to Go—Theme and Variations

You can't expect to lose weight until you are eating on demand nearly all the time—until you eat when you're hungry, eat *exactly* what your body wants, and *stop eating precisely when you are full.* The more exact you are about your body's food needs, the closer you will get to your natural weight.

Given that you are able to eat on demand, however, it's hard to predict precisely how your weight loss will progress and how you will react to it.

Leveling Off: We have found over the years that when most people eat on demand, they lose some weight, then level off for a time before they lose some more. Sometimes this means that you drop several pounds and gain back a few. This sort of leveling off is natural. Radical changes of any kind are hard to assimilate. If you change too quickly you don't have the opportunity to come to terms with yourself at each stage.

People who are most successful at losing weight this gradual way are bemused when others exclaim about the weight they've lost. They know that they've changed, but because they've been looking in the mirror and accepting themselves at each stage, they don't see themselves as looking so radically different.

Pushing Yourself: This slow pace can be frustrating for chronic dieters who are accustomed to the "high" that usually follows a weight loss. In our experience, people who have watched their weight most intensely in the past tend to forget that they're trying to watch their eating and accept their weight, whatever it might be.

Jennifer is eating more and more out of stomach hunger. She's thrilled with her new way of eating and decides, just for the hell of it, to step on the scale to see if anything is happening with her weight. When she looks down at the numbers and sees that she has lost five pounds she thinks, "Oh good, if I keep this up, I'll be able to fit into last year's summer clothes by next month." Strangely enough, over the next few days her eating is not quite on target, and by the end of the week, she has regained the five pounds. She is surprised and distressed. What happened?

A number of things occurred the moment Jennifer looked at the numbers on the scale. First, in a very subtle way her excitement at having lost weight was undermining. By getting so excited and thinking about losing even more weight she was actually telling herself that she wasn't okay at her current size and that she had been more unacceptable before she lost those five pounds. As Jennifer learned to feed herself on demand, she also learned to live with herself in an accepting way. When she stepped on the scale and rejoiced at her weight loss, she returned momentarily to her old judgmental self, which proclaimed fat as bad and thin as good. As soon as Jennifer told herself she was "better" at five pounds less, she rebelled against her self-imposed unacceptance and began to eat until she regained the weight.

Second, as soon as Jennifer began calculating how much weight she might lose by the summer, she was jumping ahead of her experience. We've talked about the cumulative effects of feeding oneself on demand, that each feeding experience builds on the one that it follows. Jennifer has had enough experiences of consistently feeding herself on demand in an attuned way to see a weight change. But when she imagines herself thinner, she is imagining herself many eating experiences ahead of where she is.

Remember that each time you eat on demand you are, in a subtle way, transforming yourself into a more secure person who can confront feelings and experiences without running to food. People who don't run to food with their feelings usually lose weight. You can't sustain a smaller size, however, until you are able to deal with your internal life without eating.

Jennifer clearly was not ready to think about herself in a thinner future. She needs to eat her way to that point of thinness. By imagining herself even thinner, Jennifer moved too far away from what was familiar. Her experience was similar to that of young children separating from their mothers. They crawl away quite independently, then check back to be sure their mothers are still there. Occasionally a toddler loses sight of her mother and gets frightened or upset. When she's reunited, she's apt to cling and stay close until she feels secure enough about her mother's presence to separate again.

Jennifer saw that she had lost weight and put herself pounds ahead of where she was ready to be. In response, she had to move back to a comfortable level.

We appreciate the temptation to become excited about a weight loss and project into the future. There is a real difference, however, between being pleased about your accomplishments and being judgmental. It is terrific that your body is responding to your noncompulsive eating. It is thrilling to see that you can lose weight without dieting and self-hatred. But you must guard against the kind of excitement that derives from a lack of self-acceptance of yourself as you are or as you were at your largest.

Holding On to Yourself: We said that some of you may discover that even though your eating has changed radically, your size has not. Those of you who sense that your natural weight could be still lower, that your failure to lose weight is not a result of metabolic or genetic factors, may simply need more time and practice with demand feeding. It may be that despite the changes in your eating, you still need to use food as a soother often enough to prevent weight loss. As you make progress in breaking your addiction to food, you can expect your weight to change.

Others of you may eat from mouth hunger infrequently

but do it just enough to maintain the status quo rather than lose weight. You may eat just a bit beyond fullness or you may not always be precise about when and what to eat. Weight loss occurs when you eat exactly when, what, and how much your body dictates.

If you sense that you are reluctant to be that precise, you might ask yourself some questions. Do you eat beyond fullness because you haven't developed a sense of what constitutes fullness? Is food still "charged" for you, and does that charge make it difficult to leave it behind? Or is it possible that your unwillingness to be precise about your eating results from your reluctance to see the changes in your eating behavior reflected in your body size?

We are consistently surprised by people's reactions to changes in their body size. People come to us because they want to lose weight, and when they hear what we have to say, they become interested in the question of their addiction to food. They set about solving that problem, and as they do, they become more accepting of themselves and more knowledgeable about the issues that they struggle with in their lives. But some of these people seem to hold on to their weight. When we explore the causes, we discover that they are more reluctant to part with their weight than one would imagine.

You may have heard it said that some people have an unconscious need to be fat or, conversely, that people have fears about being thin. What this means is that being fat or being thin has significance for them beyond their awareness. Susie Orbach and others have written extensively about the multiple meanings body size has for women in particular. It seems that just as we do with food, we invest the size of our bodies with magical powers. Much as we may dislike our "large" bodies, they often symbolize much that we respect—power, presence, strength, earthiness, and substance.

The Food/Fat Connection

You now know that particular situations, thoughts, or feelings have prompted you to turn to food in the past. For most of you this compulsive reach for food has resulted in either a "fat" body or the feeling that you are fat. You did not necessarily eat to make yourself fat. You ate compulsively to ward off the anxiety that was triggered by your core issues. Once you ate, however, your fatness, imagined or real, took on a life of its own.

When you are fat or think of yourself as fat, you feel culturally unacceptable, out of size and consequently out of step. We've talked about how we all internalize our culture's values and think of fat as bad and thin as good. At the same time, however, something of which we are entirely unaware is going on. Indeed, we all have associations to fat and thin that, when we first learn of them, are quite startling. Your associations to the states of fatness and thinness bear a direct relationship to the concerns that caused you to seek comfort through food.

For example, imagine that someone you care deeply about is gravely ill. You're anxious and turn to food in an attempt to ward off your feelings of loss. Regardless of whether or not you actually gain weight as a result of this kind of eating, we ask you to imagine yourself fatter and think about how you'd feel. Much to your surprise, you'll probably discover that your feelings about being bigger are not entirely bad. It may be that in your fantasy of having a larger body you actually feel safer or more protected. If, at that point, you stop and imagine yourself becoming much thinner, you may discover that you feel cold and alone. Many of us who attribute magical powers to food also attribute magical powers to our body size.

On a rational level we know that neither food nor fat can protect us from loss. If you start out feeling overwrought, you could eat and gain weight and still feel overwrought. Fatness and thinness in and of themselves do not do anything for us. They are simply a matter of physical size. However, we often cling to fat and fear being thin because of the fantasies we attach to these different body states.

Learning to understand the meanings you bring to "fat" and "thin" can help you in two ways. First, it's yet another way to learn about your real feelings. Second, if you ever hope to return to your natural weight, you must first divest fatness and thinness of their hidden meanings and regard them as sizes. Until you can see them as variations in physical size, you'll hold on to the fear that you will be losing something other than weight as you begin to shed pounds. As long as you attach fantasies to being thin, you'll have to worry about whether you can handle a "thin" life.

We ask the people in our groups to work with their fantasies to discover the hidden meanings they give to states of fatness and thinness, and we ask you to do the same.

Friendly Fat Fantasies

Imagine yourself becoming considerably heavier than you are. Although you may resist seeing yourself this way, try to allow the fantasy. Once you see and feel yourself growing larger, try to visualize precisely where you are. What's happening there? What are you doing and feeling?

Although it may seem strange to you, pretend for a moment that your fat is your friend, that it is doing something helpful for you. Try to discover precisely how your fat serves you. Assume that whatever function fat performs for you in this fantasy, whether or not you approve of it, is necessary. As you prepare to leave the fantasy, try to think of ways you could do for yourself what the fat does.

Let us give you some examples of what people we work with discover about the magic they attribute to a larger body.

Doing versus Sitting: "I hated the idea of getting heavier," said Connie, "but was I surprised. I started to feel very powerful, like one of those matriarchs in the Bible. I imagined everyone coming to me for advice, as if I were the community wise woman. Along with being wise and having great influence, I noticed that in my fantasy I barely moved at all. I just sat in one place and everyone came to me. That feeling was wonderful. I really loved never having to move or exert myself physically. I saw myself getting larger and larger and more and more stationary.

"It's odd," Connie concluded, "that someone who hates being heavy as much as I do could enjoy it as I did in my fantasy. I loved the sense of stillness and I loved the power of it. I can see how if I think of my fat in those terms I'd be reluctant to give it up."

The feelings about fat that surfaced in Connie's fantasy are not unusual. She became aware of a wish not to exert herself. In reality, Connie is a woman who makes great demands on herself, and her fantasy of not having to move is a welcome luxury. Many compulsive eaters are unaware of the extent to which they wish they could "not do." Connie's fantasy was an expression of that as well as her wish to be sought out and regarded as powerful and influential.

Understandably, for many people fat symbolizes the attainment of adulthood and the ability to be in charge. When we were children, adults seemed very large to us, very powerful and entirely in charge. Although we understand logically that we are adults by virtue of age, not girth, feelings of powerlessness often bring us back, on an emotional level, to our childhood. That's how it was with Connie.

She learned from her fantasy that when she feels powerless and least in control, she sees fat much as she did when she was a child. Since Connie is forever trying to live up to her own strict standards of how much she should accomplish, she often pushes herself way past fatigue in order to accomplish more. She never acknowledges her wishes to do nothing or her desire to be admired without having to earn the admiration.

The enormous strain of living up to her own standards is the issue that often triggers the anxiety which brings Connie to food. Resolving such a conflict is a long-term project, and Connie may need professional help along the way. In the meantime, however, she has to be able to separate that conflict from her eating and from her weight. She needs to understand that whether she's fat or thin, she will have her conflict until she deals with it head-on and resolves it. If Connie continues to explore the fantasied meaning she attributes to fat, she will be able to see her size more and more as an objective reality. And once she does that, she will be able to allow it to change.

The Triumph of Fat versus the Submission of Thin: Rima's fantasy had less detail than Connie's, but it was equally illuminating. In her fantasy, Rima kept growing larger and larger, and as she did she laughed louder and louder, more and more out of control. The laughter, Rima came to understand, had to do with a feeling of triumph. "I felt in my fantasy," she explained to the group, "that I had won out over all the people who hound me about losing weight."

Rima's fantasy came as no surprise to her. Over the course of the last year she had become an excellent demand feeder, and during that year she had begun to shed her weight several times. Yet each time the weight loss became noticeable, something triggered a compulsive return to food and fat.

"Every time I lose weight someone comes over to me and says how fabulous I look," Rima explained, "and the next thing I know is that I'm eating. All I'm aware of when people compliment me is that I feel confused. I feel that I'm supposed to thank them for the compliment, but I don't want to. What kind of compliment is it anyway? They're really saying that I looked terrible before.

"I've also noticed," Rima continued, "that I sometimes have a similar response when I've lost weight and notice the weight loss in the mirror. It's as though my having lost weight is a sign of submission that I have to fight against. A few hours later I'm eating something I don't even want."

Rima's reaction to compliments on her weight loss is not unusual. Her fantasy tells the story. Rima spent a lifetime being told to lose weight. As a child she was told endlessly that she had a pretty face and "if only . . ." It's no wonder that she imagines her fat to be a triumph over all the unaccepting, oppressive, critical voices. Rima, like all of us, wants to be accepted for who she is, not for being thin or fat.

Whenever Rima loses weight she becomes confused. Is her weight loss a submission to the harsh voices of her past? Is she losing the weight for *them*? Is she losing weight to satisfy her internalized version of the harsh voices of her childhood? The rebel within Rima who has resisted all of their efforts to get her to lose weight gets nervous every time she drops a pound. "Watch out," the rebel says, "you're giving in to them."

Rima is evidently not convinced that when she loses weight as a result of demand feeding, the loss is attributable to nothing but her own needs and choices. Regarding weight loss as a submission to criticism and self-loathing, she holds on to her fat and laughs victoriously.

Before she can allow herself to lose weight, Rima needs to be certain that she accepts herself fat or thin. She must be so sure about it that when others compliment her on having become thin, when they infer that "you've become a good girl at last, haven't you?" she will not feel the need to react defiantly by gaining weight. She must understand that her weight loss is the end result of a process that has nothing to do with diets, self-loathing, or conforming to the demands of others. It has to do, instead, with self-acceptance and the ability to provide for oneself. Whether she says it out loud or not, Rima must be able to say to herself "I like the way I look now; but the way I looked before was also okay with me."

Fat Visibility: David is a person who has trouble feeling successful. He told us that he had trouble with his eating when his brother was visiting for a week. He thought that perhaps his eating problems stemmed from the feelings of competition that had always existed between him and his brother, and he was aware, during the visit, of having downplayed many of his recent accomplishments. Clearly something was going on.

In his fantasy about getting larger, David saw himself lecturing to an audience. Although the fantasy included David's feeling embarrassed about his size, he thought it was significant that he chose to fantasize about a situation in which he was the focus of attention. David has great difficulty calling attention to himself, but his wish to do so became quite evident in his fantasy.

We suggested to David that he reacts to his wish to be in the spotlight as though it were a "bad" wish, and rather than think it through, he turns to food, which is what happened during his brother's visit. Had he been able to talk about them, his recent accomplishments would have put him in the limelight, and his reluctance to be there kept David from discussing his achievements and led him to food.

In the past, David would have said that he was bad for eating, but the badness he felt really referred to his wish to be the center of attention. The truth is that David has often used his size as a rationalization for remaining on the sidelines. David's fantasy portrays his conflict very well. While he puts himself in the center of the scene, he feels embarrassed. His large size unconsciously expresses his wish to command attention and, simultaneously, his disapproval of it.

It may take David a long time to come to terms with these issues, and he, like other long-term compulsive eaters, may seek professional help in the process. But recognizing that his concern about showing off is going to be a concern whether he's fat or thin should make it easier for David to lose weight.

* * *

Once you begin to understand what function "fat" serves for you, you will be in a position to separate that wish from your fat. Remember that fat's only properties are the ones you give it.

Thinness in and of itself also means nothing. Although we've talked about how society equates "thin" with "good," you'll be surprised to discover that you attribute many different meanings to the state of being thin, not all of them positive.

The Fear of Thinness

Our group work with thin fantasies is much like that with fat fantasies.

Imagine yourself thin. In what scene do you envision yourself when you think of yourself as being much thinner? Look around to see what you're doing and feeling.

At first glance, this situation may seem to you like a dream come true, but think about it. What if you really did become thin and found yourself situated in your fantasy? What sorts of problems would you experience? How could you resolve those problems without regaining your weight?

Once you begin to explore these fantasies, it becomes clear that, just as fat is not all bad, thinness is not all good. Here are some typical reactions to the fantasy of being thin.

Invisibility: Margot told the group about the hard time she had getting an image of herself thin. "But then I tried to feel myself getting thinner bit by bit, and I could picture it. The problem was that the process of getting thinner in my fantasy just wouldn't stop," Margot explained. "First, I looked weak and fragile, almost childlike. It was hardly a good situation. I looked gaunt. But then I had the thought that I would simply disappear. It was strange and frightening. I know that I exist whether I'm thin or fat, so why would I think of myself disappearing?"

Margot's fear is a common one among compulsive eaters. Food and weight are equated in their minds with strength and substance. The evening that Margot described her fantasy, she had been talking about some trouble she'd been having with mouth hunger. She'd been successfully feeding herself on demand for some time, but during the last few days she noticed that she'd been eating more and more from mouth hunger. She traced the trouble to having been passed over earlier that week for a promotion she thought was in the bag. She felt overlooked, but she was also embarrassed about having been so certain that the promotion would be hers.

Margot's mouth hunger was strongly connected to her fantasy of being thin. She was having trouble holding on to her sense of herself as a significant person in the face of what she considered a rejection. In her fantasy of being thin, Margot disappears. She loses her very existence. Thin, in her fantasy, means invisible. What can Margot do?

In our experience, this equation between becoming thin and being small and childlike is as common as the equation between being fat and being an adult. Our confusion between childlike and thin feeds into the fantasy of disappearing or becoming insignificant. Margot feels slighted and overlooked in the workplace. As a child she may have had similar feelings of being unable to make an impact. But Margot's feelings about having been passed over and those from her childhood have nothing, in reality, to do with her body size.

On Display: Jill imagined herself walking into a lavish party. "I looked fabulous," she said, "so great that all eyes were on me. It was hard for me to think of any problems in the fantasy. It seemed nice to be getting the attention. If I think about it, though, I guess if I ever really got that much attention I'd probably worry about how other people felt about it. I'd be concerned that I was taking the attention away from someone else or that people would envy me."

When compulsive eaters imagine themselves thin, they often imagine themselves on display. We all share the wish to show ourselves off or show what we can do, but many of us feel guilty about our desires. Yet we have them, and the question is what to do about them. Fat ought not to mean that we have to hide, and thin ought not to mean that we automatically start to parade around.

We have to decide what makes us comfortable or uncomfortable vis-à-vis display. There are ways of taking the spotlight or avoiding it that do not involve getting fatter or thinner. If you want to show off but are afraid to, it's important that you give yourself permission to lose weight and remain in the shadows until you're more comfortable with your size.

The Function of the Fantasy

The fantasies of becoming fatter or thinner are yet another way for you to learn something about the areas that trouble you. The point of the exercise is not necessarily to solve your problems, although knowing about them does constitute a step in that direction. The point of the exercise is to alert you to the hidden meanings you give to being fat or thin. Those meanings get in your way as you attempt to feed yourself on demand and return to your natural weight.

Essentially, you must consistently reassure yourself about two things. First, remind yourself that becoming thinner does not involve becoming younger or childlike. Check to see whether your fear of becoming thin stems from a feeling or situation you experienced in childhood, like feeling alone, helpless, shy, out of control, and so forth. Second, remind yourself that you can look different without having to do anything differently.

If you're shy and you lose weight, it's unrealistic to expect that you will become a social butterfly. If learning to socialize more comfortably is one of your goals, by all means work on it. But don't expect a change in your size to resolve the problem.

· If you enjoy attracting attention but become anxious when you get it, it doesn't make sense for you to lose weight and start wearing your most revealing clothing. You may want to attract attention, but you ought not do it without respecting the part of you that is uncomfortable in the spotlight.

Imagining that when you become thin you will become very sexually active isn't a reason for you to remain fat. Once you have separated thinness from heightened sexual activity, you will be in a position to take responsibility for determining what kind of sex life you have. You can make decisions about your behavior rather than substitute fat for decision making. If once you become thinner you have conflicts about your sexual wishes, you can think about what does and doesn't feel right for you. Wishes, after all, are not deeds.

If whenever you imagine yourself thin and attractive you

are alone, you need to think about your social life. You may have used your fat to explain why you don't have the companionship you desire, but you need to own up to loneliness as a problem in your life, one which will exist as much when you are thin as when you are fat until you address it directly.

As you unravel the significance you give to the states of fatness or thinness, your body will be freed to return to its natural weight. In the process, you will also have increased your knowledge about yourself. Once your body size is no longer charged with meaning, you have the opportunity to move out of an obsession and into real life.

Afterword

"How long does it take to do all this?" "How many people have been successful with this approach?" "Will I lose weight?" Perhaps these questions are still on your mind.

All the diets you've ever followed have promised you clear results, namely weight loss within a certain time frame. Our goals are different and we make no such specific claims. However, we can say something about what to anticipate if you start feeding yourself on demand.

Your ability to use what you've read will depend on where you are in your life—whether you are ready to give up the magic of dieting and do something radically different. Each compulsive eater who embarks on this approach is charting his or her own course. You will choose when to eat, what to eat, and how much to eat. Your eating will bear the stamp of your unique signature.

Some people hear this material once, stop dieting, set up their new eating system, and break the addictive circuit within months. They may backslide occasionally; they may eat just enough to maintain their weight if they fear losing it; they may begin to lose weight or they may discover that their natural weight is not as far from their current one as they thought. In any case, they're out of the woods. But most people require more time and must relearn the concepts again and again before they are able to incorporate them in their lives. Remember that you are striving to create a new system out of an old, entrenched one.

You are, in effect, struggling to *cure* a problem that you thought you'd have to *control* forever. What everyone who takes a chance on giving up food restrictions discovers is that life can be radically different from anything they could have anticipated. Their compulsive need for food diminishes greatly, and with time and effort, it can cease altogether.

The initial questions people pose about success pertain to weight loss. Before long, however, they develop new measures of progress. For a compulsive eater to live comfortably in a house well stocked with food, to binge no longer, to remain at a constant weight which, in time, goes down slowly, and to have more and more time free from obsessive thoughts about eating and weight are major accomplishments that were formerly unimaginable. Ultimately, the loss of pounds is a pleasure, a side effect and fringe benefit of the profound alteration in the quality of people's lives.

Remind yourself as you begin this approach that demand feeding is an act of self-assertion. Each time you eat from stomach hunger you are taking care of yourself in a direct way. As you begin to do this more and more, you will feel better about yourself and increasingly able to handle the issues that confront you in life.

We wish you all good luck and bon appetit!

Supplementary Reading

Many books have been published on the topic of compulsive eating and overweight. We have selected those which we feel will be most helpful to you in moving forward with our approach.

Bennett, William, M.D., and Gurin, Joel. *The Dieter's Dilemma*. New York: Basic Books, 1982.

Bilich, Marion. *Weight Loss from the Inside Out: Help for the Compulsive Eater*. New York: Harper & Row, 1983.

Chernin, Kim. *The Obsession: Reflections on the Tyranny of Slenderness*. New York: Harper & Row, 1981.

Hirschmann, Jane R., and Zaphiropoulos, Lela. *Are You Hungry? A Completely New Approach to Raising Children Free of Food and Weight Problems*. New York: New American Library, 1987.

Kaplan, Louise. *Oneness and Separateness: From Infant to Individual*. New York: Simon and Schuster, 1978.

Orbach, Susie. *Fat Is a Feminist Issue*, New York: Berkley, 1978.

———. *Fat Is a Feminist Issue II*. New York: Berkley, 1982.

———. *Hunger Strike*. New York: Norton, 1987.

Polivy, Janet, and Herman, C. Peter. *Breaking the Diet Habit*. New York: Basic Books, 1983.

Roberts, Nancy. *Breaking All the Rules*. New York: Viking, 1986.

Roth, Geneen. *Feeding the Hungry Heart*. New York: Signet, 1983.

———. *Breaking Free from Compulsive Eating*. New York: Signet, 1986.

Siegel, Michele, Brisman, Judith, Weinshel, Margot. *Surviving an Eating Disorder: New Perspectives and Strategies for Family and Friends*. New York: Harper & Row, 1988.

Index

More Books from Vermilion

Prices correct at time of going to press

If you have enjoyed this book you might like these titles from Vermilion:

To order your copies from Vermilion
(P&P free) call
TBS DIRECT on **01206 255800.**

The authors can be contacted at:
Overcoming Overeating
P.O. Box 1257,
Old Chelsea Station,
New York, New York 10011